Drugs in Perspective

DRUGS IN PERSPECTIVE

Martin A. Plant
BSc, MA, PhD

Senior Research Fellow, Alcohol Research Group,
Department of Psychiatry, University of Edinburgh

HODDER AND STOUGHTON
LONDON   SYDNEY   AUCKLAND   TORONTO

British Library Cataloguing in Publication Data

Plant, Martin A.
  Drugs in perspective.
  1. Drugs – Physiological effect
  I. Title
  615'.7   RM300

  ISBN 0 340 40149 4

First published 1981 as *Teach Yourself Drugs in Perspective*
First published in this edition 1987

Copyright © 1987 Martin A. Plant

No part of this publication may be reproduced or transmitted in any form or by any means, electronically or mechanically, including photocopying, recording or any information storage or retrieval system, without either the prior permission in writing from the publisher or a licence, permitting restricted copying, issued by the Copyright Licensing Agency, 7 Ridgmount Street, London WC1E 7AA.

Typeset in Plantin by
Rowland Phototypesetting Ltd,
Bury St Edmunds, Suffolk

Printed and bound in Great Britain for
Hodder and Stoughton Educational,
a division of Hodder and Stoughton Ltd,
Mill Road, Dunton Green, Sevenoaks, Kent
by Richard Clay Ltd, Bungay, Suffolk

Contents

Acknowledgements	vii
Figures and tables	ix
Preface	xi
1 The Background	1
2 Drugs and Their Effects	12
3 Why People Use Drugs	32
4 Drugs and the Law	45
5 Patterns of Drugtaking	58
6 Drug Problems	83
7 What Becomes of Drugtakers?	118
8 What Can Be Done?	127
9 Conclusions	140
Appendix I Some useful Addresses	142
Appendix II Some recommended reading/Bibliography	157
Index	171

This book is dedicated to Moira and Emma

Acknowledgements

The preparation of this book was assisted by many people and agencies. A considerable amount of the material presented stems from countless unrecorded conversations with colleagues concerned with research into drug use and misuse or the provision of services to help those with drug problems. Many of the sources that helped to form the perspective of this book are not cited. Invaluable help, advice and information were obtained from the following people: Professor H. Ross Anderson, Mr Mike Ashton, Dr Ifti Akhter, Dr Dorothy Black, Mr David Chambers, Dr Alex Crawford, Dr Elizabeth Crofton, Dr Phil Davies, Dr Jim Dyer, Dr Cindy Fazey, Ms Pam Gillies, Dr Hamid Ghodse, Professor Norman Kreitman, Professor Malcolm Lader, Dr Frank Ledwith, Ms Joy Mott, Mr David Peck, Dr Bruce Ritson, Dr Roy Robertson, Dr Anthony Thorley, Mr Christopher Thurman and Dr Laurence Whalley. In addition, information was kindly made available to the author by the following agencies: Alcohol Concern, Action on Smoking and Health (ASH), the Advertising Association, the Brewers' Society, the Department of Health and Social Security, The Guardian, the Home Office, the Institute for the Study of Drug Dependence, the Office of Population Censuses and Surveys, the Medical Council on Alcoholism, the Scotch Whisky Association, the Scottish Committee of ASH, the Scottish Health Education Group, the Scottish Home and Health Department, the Tobacco Advisory Council, the Welsh Office and Yellowhammer PLC.

Dr Moira Plant read the initial draft of the text and suggested sensible improvements. Mrs Ray Stuart assisted with the compilation of the list of useful addresses and the bibliography. The typing was efficiently carried out by Mrs Janis Nichol. The defects of this book are, of course, solely the author's responsibility.

March 1987   Martin Plant

Figures and Tables

Figures

2.1 Units of alcohol
8.1 It's all the same to your liver
8.2 No wonder smokers cough
8.3 Smoking gets right up other people's noses
8.4 Heroin screws you up
8.5 Choose life, not drugs

Tables

4.1 Misuse of Drugs Act (1971). Offences and maximum penalties.
5.1 Per capita alcohol consumption in twenty six countries (1950 and 1983).
5.2 Average alcohol consumption in the United Kingdom.
5.3 Prevalence of cigarette smoking among males aged sixteen and over in Britain (1972–1982).
5.4 Prevalence of cigarette smoking among females aged sixteen and over in Britain (1972–1982).
5.5 Cigarette consumption of people aged sixteen and over in Britain (1972–1982).
5.6 Prevalence of cigarette smoking in Britain by age and sex (1972–1984).
5.7 Percentage of current cigarette smokers in Scotland and three English regions (1976).
5.8 Regional variations in self-reported illicit drug use amongst the 15–21 age group in Britain.
5.9 Changes in self-reported drug use amongst a study group of young people in the Lothian Region (1979/80 to 1983).
5.10 Drugs ever used by regular illicit drugtakers in two British studies.
5.11 Barbiturate prescriptions in Britain (1972–1984).
5.12 Benzodiazepine prescriptions in Britain (1980 and 1984).

6.1 Recent trends in alcohol consumption and alcohol-related problems in the United Kingdom.
6.2 Liver cirrhosis mortality amongst British males in different occupations (1979–80, 1982–83).
6.3 Rates of liver cirrhosis mortality in twenty five countries (1983).
6.4 Age distribution of those aged 35–64 dying of tobacco-related diseases (United Kingdom) (1977).
6.5 Mortality from malignant neoplasms of trachea, bronchus and lung amongst British men in different occupations (1979–80, 1982–83).
6.6 Rates of lung cancer mortality in twenty four countries (1955–1975).
6.7 Number of seizures of controlled drugs (1974–1984).
6.8 Persons found guilty of drug offences (1979–84).
6.9 Narcotic drug addicts known to the Home Office (1970–1984).
6.10 Age distribution of narcotic drug addicts known to the Home Office at 31 December 1984.
6.11 Type of drugs prescribed to notified addicts during 1984.
6.12 Drugs ever taken 'for kicks' by seventy two Scottish hospital attenders.

Preface

As the title suggests, this book is an attempt to present the use and misuse of psychoactive (mind altering) drugs in a balanced and rational way. During the past two to three decades enormous attention has been paid to 'the problem' of recreational drug experimentation by young people, to 'alcoholism' and to the health hazards inherent in tobacco smoking. At the same time growing concern has been voiced at the increasing levels at which mood altering drugs are prescribed (or over-prescribed) by medical practitioners.

The author, a sociologist, initially began research into the use and misuse of illegal drugs such as cannabis, LSD and heroin. Subsequently he became primarily concerned with research into the use of alcohol and its related problems. This dual experience led to the form of this book, which relates not only to the much publicised use of spectacular or illegal drugs by young people, but also to society's legal 'acceptable' drugs, alcohol and tobacco, and to drugs taken on medical prescription. It is a principal contention of this book that it is often misleading to consider drugs only as 'legal' or 'illegal'. A more realistic and complete assessment requires information about the properties of the substance, the characteristics of the user and the context of use. Most psychoactive drugs can sometimes be taken in moderation and without harm. All can be misused or may give rise to problems, even tragedies, if taken inappropriately or excessively. Far too often the legal drugs, alcohol and tobacco, have been treated as if they are much safer than, and altogether different from, illegal or prescribed substances. This is not necessarily so and a huge amount of common ground exists between the literatures and debates related to, on the one hand, alcohol and tobacco and, on the other hand, illegal substances such as cannabis, LSD and heroin. This book attempts to discuss psychoactive drugs in general and, where appropriate, to draw parallels and present overall conclusions. It is not suggested, of course, that the illegal use of cannabis by young people is precisely the same sort of thing as the legal use of alcohol or tobacco. Even so, it is stressed that the many different types of drug-related behaviour can be considered in general terms. The evidence about why people use drugs and what happens to these people is strikingly similar in relation to both legal and illegal drugs.

In addition, ideas of what constitutes 'addiction' or 'drug dependence' and conclusions about what becomes of dependent individuals also appear similar in relation to legal and illegal drugs.

This book describes the effects, patterns of use and problems related to the general range of psychoactive drugs. The issues of social acceptability and legality are discussed in relation to the evidence of the relative safety, danger and effects of the most commonly used or misused substances. It is hoped that the information presented here will assist those requiring an up-to-date summary of some of the extensive drug literature and debate. In addition, it is intended that this book will provide a source of factual information for those engaged in the 'helping professions' – doctors, nurses, psychologists, social workers and others who require a straightforward account of practical issues such as the effects of specific drugs, details of drug-related harm, what becomes of drugtakers and information about providing help for those who require it.

In order to facilitate easier reading very few references are cited directly in the text. Standard 'academic' procedure would be to support every statement with specific references. This omission is partially compensated for by presenting a select list of recommended reading in Appendix II as well as an extensive bibliography.

From the perspective presented in this book it is hoped that the reader will conclude that many reasons appear to explain why varied types of drug use occur and that drug users and misusers do not conform to the popularly accepted stereotypes. In view of the diversity both of reasons for and patterns of drug use, it emerges that drug-related problems are unlikely to be countered by any single approach. In addition, the effectiveness of many popular activities such as health education campaigns are sometimes intangible, disappointing or only evident in the long-term. Much drug use is casual and harmless, and is certainly pleasant if not beneficial. The force and perils of physical dependence upon substances such as heroin have often been greatly exaggerated and problems with legal or illegal drugs are neither necessarily incurable nor do they in themselves constitute a disease.

1 The Background

Drug use in some form or other is virtually universal. This is not new. The earliest writings refer to the use of opium, cannabis and alcohol and it is almost certain that such substances were used by humans long before they became literate. To a large extent, the types of drugs used and favoured by each social group have been a matter of botanical and geographical convenience. People have generally sought a change of consciousness with the aid of whatever appropriate vegetation or other source was available. Alcohol, humanity's 'oldest drug', is the most widely used because it can be produced from the fermentation of so many types of plant. The near universality of drug use has even prompted the suggestion that the propensity to use drugs is what distinguishes humans from other animals.

During the twentieth century, 'drug misuse' has become widely regarded as one of society's great problems. It is abundantly clear that all over the world various types of drugs are increasingly being used excessively, unwisely and often harmfully. At the same time the pharmaceutical industry is producing an almost unbelievable range of new drugs to meet the ever growing demand for substances that can allay depression and anxiety, dull pain, stimulate or aid sleep. Humanity has a love-hate relationship with drugs. They inspire awe, fear and even lust. The complexity of the situation has been perceptively described by Professor Griffith Edwards:

'If you were to fly low over any part of the earth's land surface, you would have a fair chance of before long seeing below you some process of drug cultivation. You would see vineyards, coffee plantations, wide areas where the tobacco crop shaped the economy, fields of opium poppy, patches of lank Indian hemp flowering even on vacant city lots. The coca plant grows on the slopes of the Andes, so that six million peasants shall obtain their cocaine. Even the desert has the peyote cactus. As you looked down on the great industrial countries it would be the factories, however, rather than the fields which would properly catch your attention: modern technology spills out its tranquillisers, stimulants, analgesics and antidepressants by the billions, and the chemist much improves on cactus and mushroom.

You would know that everywhere below varieties of actors were in the arena, and with extraordinary changeability of roles. Sometimes the state would sell the drug and take the profit, sometimes the profit would go to the legally operating entrepreneur, sometimes that role would be played by the man with the mule train who makes his way over the mountain paths. The money at stake is immense and countries might finance their treasuries to a large extent from drug revenues. Conflicts of opinion are violent, the state's response to unpermitted use draconian. The situation on which you looked down would, however, seem to be characterised by an unusual degree of confusion: a drug which was permissible yesterday might tomorrow be prohibited; a drug which for one society was of importance in religious sacrament might in another place be preached against. You could conclude that one of the main businesses of the world was to cultivate, manufacture, advertise, legislate on, tax, consume, adulate and decry mind-acting substances. The complexity of the matter is overwhelming, its ramifications endless.' (Edwards 1971)

As noted in the Preface, this book is not only concerned with exotic, illegal substances that 'deviant', disaffected young people use to evade reality or responsibility. Nor is it concerned solely with the 'misuse' or harmful use of drugs. It is intended that the following pages will describe at least some of the main aspects of both 'normal' and less commonplace drug use, both in relation to legal and illegal substances. Such general coverage is important for two main reasons. First, one cannot realistically appreciate either the causes of drug-related problems or devise likely solutions to them unless one considers by whom, why and when drugs are generally used. Secondly, while youthful drug misuse is justifiably a cause for concern in many countries, the great majority of drug-related damage is caused by tobacco smoking and by the misuse of alcohol or of prescribed drugs, often taken by middle-aged or elderly people. It is unrealistic to pretend that alcohol, tobacco, Librium, Valium and Ativan are not drugs or that, because their use is legal, they cannot produce dependence or other problems. Conversely, it does not follow that simply because cannabis, LSD, heroin and other substances are proscribed for recreational use, they are necessarily inherently more 'addictive' or harmful than some of the widely accepted legal drugs.

Some popular stereotypes and misconceptions

Public thinking about 'the drug problem' is highly coloured by lurid media coverage which often exaggerates and sensationalises both the scale and meaning of various forms of drug use. There is little doubt that popular thinking about drug-related problems is often influenced by extreme and oversimple stereotypes. The 'drug pusher', for example, must rank as high (or as low?) in the twentieth century demonology as the paedophile. It has been very widely accepted that many young people are somehow 'lured' into drugtaking and thereby on to the rocks of drug dependence by the malevolent seductions of commercial drug traders. Such a view has been ardently fostered both by the popular press, by television dramatisations and sometimes by well-meaning authorities such as politicians, the clergy or the police. In fact, as described in Chapters 3 and 5, this view appears to be grossly inaccurate, or at least an oversimple and myopic explanation, of why so many young people have begun to experiment with illegal drugs.

The popularly accepted image of the 'drugtaker' is of a dirty, long-haired social derelict injecting himself or herself into an early grave. Similarly, the 'alcoholic' is also widely perceived to be destitute, although older, typically imbibing 'meths', Brasso or other improbable beverages while sleeping rough or 'skippering' among disused buildings. There is no doubt that some drug misusers are beset by a great many problems. Some are jobless, homeless and bereft. Some do kill themselves. The majority do not and cannot be so neatly consigned to such simple (and comfortingly remote) categories.

As the following chapters will attempt to clarify, both drug users and drug misusers are enormously varied. They simply do not conform to any uniform patterns. This is as true of those who use illegal drugs as it is of tobacco smokers or alcohol drinkers. In addition, it is now clear from a considerable body of evidence that most people who suffer harmful consequences from their particular types of drug use are not, as is so often supposed, a race apart from the majority of other drug users, whose use appears to be harmless or at least generally passes unnoticed by 'official agencies' such as the police or medical services.

Traditional popular ideas about illegal drug misuse owe a great deal to propaganda designed to frighten people away from experimenting with illegal substances such as cannabis. In addition, such propaganda has often circulated generalisations about illegal drug use based upon highly atypical individuals such as heroin injectors in clinics. In consequence, it has often been stressed that everyone who uses illegal drugs runs a high risk of becoming physically dependent upon such substances or that such drug use implies some deep-seated psychological defects. It has been uncritically accepted that those who use illegal drugs are by definition flawed personalities, inadequate or in some way 'suitable for treatment'. At the same time, it has been suggested that the use of illegal drugs is a different type of phenomenon from the more mundane use of alcohol, tobacco or prescribed drugs.

'I smoke tobacco, but I would never use drugs. They frighten me.'

This comment was made to the author by an intelligent colleague during the preparation of this book. These sentiments are by no means uncommon either among the general public or even among professionals who daily help those with drug problems.

While it is generally conceded that the harmful consequences of tobacco use or of excessive drinking are a serious cause for concern, these are seldom discussed as part of a more general pattern of drug misuse. Alcohol problems are often portrayed in a way that sets them apart from the experiences of most drinkers. The most influential force on recent public thinking about drinking problems has been the self-help organisation Alcoholics Anonymous (AA). The central beliefs of AA are that 'alcoholics' are basically people who are, by their constitutional makeup, 'allergic' to alcohol. They have a disease which is incurable and which may only be countered by perpetual abstinence. In fact, these views are tenets of faith. They are not the outcome of scientific inquiry and they are not consistent with a considerable body of evidence about drinking problems that has been produced during the past thirty years. AA has done, and continues to accomplish, a very great deal of good work in encouraging some problem drinkers to abstain. In addition, AA has probably helped to create a much more humane and constructive climate of opinion wherein drinking problems can be helped. However, one consequence of the well-known AA view that 'alcoholism' is an incurable disease is that problem drinkers continue to be generally regarded as wholly different from other alcohol users. Just as the illegal drugtaker has been effectively segregated from the rest of humanity in the public mind, so has the problem drinker. In fact, there is a continuum of people using all manner of drugs. Most take things sensibly, cautiously and in moderation. A minority use drugs heavily and some become dependent or suffer other forms of harm. This is as true of the legal drugs as it is of the illegal ones. The picture is further confused by what has been called the 'preventive paradox'. The relative risk that a person will experience drug-related harm is much higher if that person is a heavy or chronic user. Even so, most drug-related problems involve people who are relatively moderate users simply because such people vastly outnumber those who are very heavy or dependent users.

It is by no means true that, because somebody uses an illegal drug, that person is particularly likely to become either physically dependent or seriously damaged thereby. Neither is it a probability or even a great risk that casual experimentation with so-called 'soft' drugs such as cannabis will lead, by some 'stepping stone process', to deep and tragic involvement with 'hard' or dependence-producing substances such as heroin. It has long been accepted, due to the popularity of alcohol use, that moderate drinking is unlikely to lead to dependence or serious harm. In addition it is generally acknowledged that drinkers vary enormously and that most do not appear to suffer as a result of alcohol consumption, but are probably the better for it. Similar conclusions are as valid for other forms of drug use. Legal drugtakers are now clearly shown to be an extremely varied group, most of whom appear not to be harmed by their drug use. It is equally clear that many illegal drugtakers, however dubious their claims may be, are forthright in asserting that they do derive benefits from their drug use.

As Professor Griffith Edwards has cogently pointed out, the relationship between drugs and society is a confusing and complicated one. Different societies have diametrically opposed views about which substances are acceptable and which are taboo. In Islamic countries alcohol is shunned with the same vehemence as are cannabis or heroin in Britain. Different countries have had widely varied drug policies at different historical times. Drug problems have also been viewed in a wide variety of ways during different periods. Excessive drinking, for example, has been variously regarded as a moral or spiritual defect, a deplorable weakness, as a disease (and thereby deserving sympathy) and more recently as a response to social, cultural and economic pressures. Opiate dependence was regarded as a purely medical problem so long as it related to unobtrusive 'therapeutic addicts' including many doctors and nurses. A radical reappraisal occurred once opiate use was adopted by young people who combined it with a distaste for conventional values and who paraded their drug use as part of a general rejection of most of the beliefs which their parents held dear.

Moral Panics

The emergence of youthful drug misuse has attracted an enormous amount of media and scientific interest. The importation of many (originally American) drug fashions into Britain and other countries gave rise to understandable fears that the American scale of drug problems would be replicated. Throughout the 1960s and subsequently, the media have responded to evidence of new fads in teenage drug use (amphetamines, Chinese heroin, cannabis, psychedelics, alcohol, glues, Angel Dust, Iranian heroin, alcohol and back to heroin to name but a few) with almost unrivalled zeal. At the same time, relatively little attention has been paid to the fact that an estimated 100,000 people are dying in Britain each year from the direct effects of tobacco smoking. The vast media coverage of illegal drugtaking by young people is due to the fact that such behaviour has been combined with new lifestyles which, to the older generation at least, appear alien and possibly menacing. Rampant hedonism is both fascinating and sinister. The sociologist Stanley Cohen described the creation of a deviant identity thus:

'The deviant is assigned to a role or social type, shared perspectives develop through which he and his behaviour are visualized and explained, motives are inspected, causal patterns are searched for and the behaviour is grouped with other behaviour thought to be of the same order.' (Cohen 1972)

At times the media have paid excessive, almost voyeuristic, attention to fashions of drugtaking which are neither new nor particularly big problems. The sniffing of glues and solvents by some schoolchildren and other young people was blown up out of all proportion during the late 1970s. More recently, media concern about 'the heroin problem' has been reinvigorated by the connection of intravenous drug use with the Acquired Immune Deficiency Syndrome (AIDS). A repeated tendency in media coverage of illegal drug use has been to infer that if a few young people are using substances (such as glues) excessively, they are necessarily typical of all those who sometimes indulge in such practices. In fact, drugtakers known to 'official agencies' are invariably far from typical. They are usually among those most deeply involved with drugs and are often beset by other major difficulties, just as problem drinkers seeking the help of treatment agencies are obviously far from typical of drinkers in general.

Another often repeated error is for the media to portray illegal drugtaking, or drug problems in general, as automatically involving 'addiction' or physical dependence. As noted above, the extent and seriousness of the risks of such dependence have been much over-emphasised. Even today some 'educational' propaganda warns people that if they use opiates they will probably become dependent:

'One fix and you're hooked.'

The message is complemented by the AA dictum that, for an 'alcoholic', a single drink will invariably suffice to revive dependence, or at least begin a binge.

'One drink, one drunk.'

In fact, it is now clear that many people use opiates intermittently for protracted periods without becoming dependent. It is also well established that some problem drinkers subsequently return to problem-free, 'social', 'moderate' or 'controlled' drinking. Different people have varied experiences with drugs.

The Paradox

Virtually every social group has its own pattern of drug use, either for purely casual, social purposes or for some more ritualised reasons. In many societies the convivial consumption of alcohol is an important part of most social gatherings. Until recently, tobacco smoking also received widespread social support although during the past few years in Britain this has steadily declined. At the same time a seemingly never-ending flow of new drugs is being marketed by the pharmaceutical industry. There is a huge and growing demand for these legally available products and most people clearly approve of, as well as indulge in, some form of drug use.

The production and distribution of alcohol, tobacco and prescribed drugs are important industries. Over 750,000 people work in the drink trade in Britain and approximately 18,000 are engaged in making tobacco products. There are over 200,000 tobacco retail outlets throughout Britain. In addition, many more people are employed in the production of medicines of various types or have jobs involving the sale or distribution of alcohol, tobacco and prescribed drugs. The Government receives enormous sums of money from the excise duty and VAT derived from alcohol and tobacco sales. During 1985 income so gained exceeded £5,700 million from alcohol and £5,000 million from tobacco. The scale of legal drug production and consumption can be further appreciated by the magnitude of the cost of advertising these commodities. In 1985 over £100 million were spent advertising alcohol and over £50 million were spent advertising tobacco products. In addition it has been estimated that British tobacco companies annually spend a further £10 million on indirect advertising, such as the sponsorship of sporting events. British television screens one hour of sport daily that is sponsored by the tobacco industry. The pharmaceutical industry too spends considerable sums on 'hospitality' for doctors, designed to promote their products. Alcohol, tobacco and prescribed drugs are big business. They constitute an important sector of manufacturing industry and generate a substantial proportion of national revenue. The dilemma resulting from the apparent importance and success of these industries is that the obvious advantages of their products are accompanied by extensive harm due to their unwise use or, in the case of tobacco, from their inherent toxicity. It is truly a paradox that the greatest drug problems of any society invariably relate to those substances which are most widely accepted and used. In the British context, this is demonstrated by the annual toll of an estimated 100,000 premature deaths due to tobacco smoking, over 200,000 drunkenness and drunken driving convictions, approximately 16,000 hospital admissions for alcohol dependence and alcoholic psychosis and the many thousands of middle-aged and elderly people who become dependent upon prescribed tranquillisers and sleeping tablets. In addition to these, many other harmful consequences related to the legal drugs are also evident. These include overdoses from alcohol or prescribed drugs (or mixtures of both), accidents while under the influence of alcohol or other substances, family disruption, violence, financial and occupational harm, and deaths from liver cirrhosis, heart disease and numerous other drug-related causes.

There is no doubt whatever that far more people are adversely affected by the legal drugs than by the illegal ones, simply because the legal ones are far more widely used. This does not, of course, imply that the legal substances are therefore more dangerous than the illegal ones. There would certainly be far more problems related to cannabis and other illegal substances if these too were in greater use. Even so, it is worth remembering that in 1984 the Home Office recorded *only* 5,869 known 'addicts' and that in 1985 *only* 26,596 people were convicted or cautioned for offences under the *Misuse of Drugs Act* (1971). Neither of these figures gives a true impression of the actual scale of illegal drug use. In spite of this, even the most liberal estimate of the extent of opiate dependence in Britain is dwarfed by the speculation that there could easily be several hundred thousand problem drinkers in the community, most of whom also produce adverse consequences for close family members or other people.

As outlined in Chapter 3, many reasons have been suggested for the existence of drug use and misuse. There is clearly a high and ever-growing demand for both alcohol and prescribed drugs and the decline in tobacco use is a recent phenomenon which may or may not be permanent. During the nineteenth and twentieth centuries many new drugs have been introduced which have revolutionised the effectiveness of medicine. Morphine, heroin and other painkillers have been of enormous therapeutic value and other drugs have transformed the management of depression and other mental disabilities. A notable consequence of the availability of the vast array of new drugs has been the extension of the role of medicine. In the past, emotional stress was regarded as being the concern of the churches. Today the most likely method of dealing with stress is medication. The increased supply of prescribed tranquillisers and sedatives is a response to growing demand for such palliatives. Many people, if not most, now visit a doctor for whatever reason in the expectation that their ailment will be treated with the appropriate medicine. Very often doctors complain that they are virtually forced into prescribing pills, tablets or potions. It is widely assumed by the public that tranquillisers or other medicines will be dispensed as a matter of course for even quite minor depression and that such substances will often be made available for protracted periods. Doctors, instead of being the arbiters of drug prescribing, sometimes find that they must respond to patients' expectations that they will receive drugs almost as a matter of right. Pressure of time in busy surgeries further enhances the appeal of a drug prescription as an expedient. It is much quicker to write such a prescription than to hold prolonged discussion of the underlying causes of anxiety or depression. Drugs, apart from their chemical properties, are symbolic. To some degree, at least, the massive level of drug prescribing reflects a popular acceptance that modern scientific medicine works primarily through drugs. It is generally acknowledged that sometimes drugs are excessively or unnecessarily prescribed, and that sometimes doctors even misunderstand the correct purpose or methods of using certain drugs. Against these shortcomings it must be emphasised that probably the overwhelming majority of prescribing of psychoactive drugs is sensible and of very great therapeutic value. In addition it is partly at least because such drugs are often so very effective that

THE BACKGROUND

the latent demand for such things has become apparent now they are available.

The technical sophistication of the twentieth century has made it possible for very many human needs to be met by the use of artificial products. If one wishes to travel, one drives, flies or takes a train. If one wishes to relax and unwind, books, music or drugs are readily available and in a hitherto unprecedented diversity. As outlined in Chapter 5, since the Second World War drinking habits in many countries have changed considerably. Alcohol consumption has risen, partly due to increased purchasing power in relation to the cost of drinks. In addition there has been an increase in leisure time and a veritable explosion of spare-time activities many of which, like hanggliding or windsurfing, are recent innovations. The role of alcohol and until recently, of tobacco, has been accordingly expanded as an adjunct to this increased time to unwind and to play. In fact, it has been suggested that the term 'addiction' should be broadened to other types of 'appetitive behaviour' with which people may become extremely or compulsively preoccupied. Gambling and sexual activity have also been described as forms of dependence, even though they are obviously qualitatively different in certain respects from dependence on psychoactive drugs.

The analogy between drug dependence and other forms of behaviour introduces an interesting insight into the way that people in minority groups prefer to be identified. An example of this is the emphasis by members of AA that they do have a disease, namely 'alcoholism'. In marked contrast most homosexuals emphatically reject any suggestion that because they are a minority, they also have a disease. Fashions change and it is important to consider who defines any form of behaviour as a problem. Research and clinical experience have shown that many people who, from some outsider's point of view, have a problem or use drugs unwisely, do not accept that this is so. This is true of thousands of people (mainly young working class males) who regularly drink to excess at weekends, of cigarette smokers in general and of those who use illegal drugs or who become dependent upon prescribed drugs. Different social groups have widely varying attitudes about which forms of drug are acceptable and which are not. While it is a major contention of this book that there are many parallels between legal and illegal drug use, there are also huge and important differences between them. Individuals have to function within their own society's values and rules. Those who do not are likely to have to face the consequences. While in some ways illegal drug use is comparable to drinking alcohol or smoking tobacco, the social reactions to these things are vastly different. An energetic vendor of alcohol or tobacco, especially an exporter of these things, might justifiably expect his or her efforts to be rewarded by a Queen's Award to British Industry. An equally energetic trader in cannabis, cocaine or heroin will be lucky to escape the official accolade of a longish prison sentence.

The social status of any particular drug depends only partly, and often to a small extent, upon its chemical properties. Most psychoactive drugs can be used in moderation under some circumstances. More important from the practical point of view is the popularity and extent of a drug's use. In particular, a decisive factor appears to be how many people in a given social group or country use a drug; a majority or a minority. In addition, it is of great significance what the dominant ideology dictates. During the past decade several Islamic countries have firmly proscribed general alcohol use. America experimented, unsuccessfully, with Prohibition and several Scandinavian countries have severely restricted the availability and price of alcoholic drinks. Recently the shift in public opinion about cigarette smoking has permitted previously inconceivable constraints upon smoking in public places. These have been much more thorough in several European countries than they have been so far in Britain, but even here a remarkable change has occurred during the past decade. Smokers are now on the defensive. The levels of restraint upon, or tolerance of, specific types of drug use reflect a largely political tolerance. If the activities of the Legalise Cannabis Campaign are some day successful, it will probably be because a majority of Members of Parliament have used the drug themselves or believe most of their constituents have done so than because a purely scientific decision has been made.

Any psychoactive drug is likely to be used unwisely, harmfully or excessively by some people. The more widely a drug is used the greater is the risk of some form of harm or misuse in relation to it. If the number of users of any drug increases, or if the average level of individual consumption rises, there will probably be more overdoses, illnesses, accidents, deaths or other catastrophes in consequence. On the other hand, increased drug use should not only be judged in relation to the problems that arise. Most people enjoy or derive some subjective, if not objective, benefits from drug use. This presumably is why drinking, smoking and other forms of drug use are so popular. It would be grossly naive and unrealistic to ignore the fact that drug use is mainly harmless, and often clearly beneficial. Most popular drugs help to reduce anxiety which in the twentieth century, beset by wars, nuclear accidents, unemployment, racialism, industrial, class and sexual conflict, is a commonplace condition.

The greatest 'drug problems' relate to the most widely used drugs. These are popular everyday products whose use is woven into our social system. Because some drugs are so popular their use is subject to relatively few constraints. Concern is expressed if their use causes harm. If anti-social behaviour ensues it will be penalised, but not the drug use itself. For this reason, alcohol use in Britain is only punished if it gets out of hand, or if people deviate markedly from the accepted norms of well-behaved, moderate drinking. Even though it is beyond dispute that tobacco smoking kills huge numbers of people, it is almost uncontrolled simply because it remains so popular and is supported by powerful vested interests. Tobacco use does

THE BACKGROUND

not of course lead to aggressive behaviour, even if it does get up other people's noses. The illegal drugs, on the other hand, have been very firmly restricted largely because their use lacks widespread public acceptance. In addition, as will be described in Chapter 4, the British social reaction to opiate use changed dramatically when this no longer involved people whose lifestyles were conventional and whose drug dependence was unobtrusive. As noted above, much of the attention and concern paid to illegal drug use by young people has been due to its association with a way of life and values that are not generally condoned.

Drug use exists in many forms and each of these needs to be considered from several aspects. Drugs vary considerably in their effects and often in relation to the doses used. Even a weak or 'safe' drug may produce strong effects or cause harmful consequences if taken in large amounts or if used inappropriately. A couple of pints of beer are usually harmless, unless one has to drive or to remain vigilant after drinking them. Even aspirins or minor tranquillisers are highly dangerous if swallowed in large numbers. The quantity and frequency in which a drug is taken are important considerations. In addition, the legal status of specific types of drug use is a major factor. As described in Chapter 4, even casual experimentation with some drugs may have extremely serious legal consequences if one is apprehended with them in one's possession. The law now lays down fairly extensive rules governing which types of drug may and may not be freely used and also goes quite a long way in restricting the supply and availability of most of the substances referred to in this book.

Drugtakers do not conform to any specific stereotype. For this reason it is fairly meaningless to assume that simply because a person has used, or is using, a certain drug that any particular consequences will necessarily ensue. Each individual case deserves separate attention. Some people do get into trouble with drugs. Most do not and this is true of both users of legal and illegal drugs. A thorough assessment of drugtaking therefore demands that several factors be considered including pharmacological, legal, social and psychological aspects of each type of drug use. Ultimately, even if considerable evidence is available, the final assessment may well be a value judgement of whether drug use is, on balance, beneficial or harmful. It is hoped that the information presented in this book will provide readers with some food for thought. In particular, it is hoped that the material presented here will, as the title suggests, help readers to consider drug use and misuse in a balanced way.

2 Drugs and Their Effects

A drug is any substance that alters the way in which the body functions. This very general definition covers a wide range of things, some of which, like antibiotics,* are normally only used on medical advice and others, such as some headache mixtures, are freely available to the general public. This book is specifically concerned with those drugs that alter the emotions or mental state. These are called *psychoactive drugs*. Alcohol and tobacco are psychoactive drugs. So are barbiturates, tranquillisers, sleeping tablets, cannabis, glues, LSD and heroin. Tea and coffee are also psychoactive drugs. These substances vary enormously both in relation to their effect on mental state and their potential dangers. Some, like LSD, are so powerful that even a single experimentation may have dramatic, sometimes tragic, results. Others, such as tobacco, do not normally produce major changes in the short-term, yet have devastatingly toxic long-term health hazards associated with their use.

There have been many attempts at classifying psychoactive drugs. A commonly used distinction has been to subdivide them into 'hard' and 'soft', depending upon whether or not they are 'addictive'. Sometimes drugs have been categorised in relation to their medical role, availability, legal status, chemical structure, mode of ingestion or in relation to their specific effects, whether they are stimulants, depressants or hallucinogens or have combinations of these effects. There is no generally agreed mode of classification and these alternatives are equally valid. In this chapter some of the basic terms and concepts of drug use and misuse are described, together with a brief indication of drug effects.

Some important terms

Regular use of some psychoactive drugs causes the body to become accustomed to their effects, which accordingly diminish. A seasoned beer drinker

* Antibiotics and similar drugs enhance the body's ability to destroy hostile invading organisms.

will, for example, learn to 'carry his or her ale'. Similarly, a person with long experience of injecting heroin may use quantities of that drug which, if taken by a novice, would be harmful or even fatal. When the body becomes so adjusted to the use of a drug, tolerance has developed. The effects of a given amount diminish so that to recapture the original experience a larger dose will be needed.

Just as the body sometimes reacts to the regular presence of a drug, it may react to a reduction or cessation of drug use. Very often such reactions are more psychological, based upon fears or expectations, than purely physical. Withdrawal symptoms, sometimes also called the abstinence syndrome, are a response to either reduction or ending of drug use once tolerance has developed. In some cases tolerance involves the body actually coming to rely upon drug use to function normally. Removal of the accustomed pattern of drug use may trigger off a physical reaction, which in the case of most drugs is slight, but which may sometimes be unpleasant or even dangerous. Withdrawal may be accompanied by stomach cramps, itching and shaking in the limbs. Drenching sweats, sleeplessness, anxiety, nausea, delirium or, in extreme cases, fits may occur. It must be emphasised that most psychoactive drugs, including heroin, do not in themselves usually produce any major withdrawal symptoms. Some of the most dramatic and dangerous withdrawal symptoms are associated not with heroin, but with alcohol and barbiturates. Usually withdrawal symptoms occur within a few hours of markedly reducing or terminating drug use. Several different terms have been used to describe such symptoms. In relation to heroin and allied drugs the experience has been called 'cold turkey'. The most extreme form of withdrawal from alcohol is called delirium tremens or the DTs. The latter appears to be rare in Britain.

The term 'addiction' is traditionally used to describe the situation when a person has to continue drug use to ward off withdrawal symptoms. This word has for some time been replaced by the term 'dependence'. This has two aspects, physical dependence and psychological dependence.

Physical dependence exists when an individual using a drug is tolerant to it and will experience physical withdrawal symptoms if usage is reduced or ended. Psychological dependence refers to an inability to function emotionally without the use of a drug. Dependence, whether physical or psychological, is not necessarily harmful. It is sometimes argued that everyone is dependent upon certain things and that sometimes such dependence is beneficial. The popular drug literature and much of the coverage of illegal drug use by the mass media have grossly over-emphasised the seriousness and extent of withdrawal from certain drugs, notably the opiates; opium, morphine, heroin and allied drugs. It is now clear that very often drug withdrawal can be accomplished relatively painlessly. In addition, many of the supposed signs of physical dependence are sometimes psychosomatic reactions triggered off not by the chemical properties of psychoactive drugs, but by the user's fears, beliefs and fantasies about what withdrawal entails.

The drugs people take

Alcohol

Alcohol is certainly the world's most widely used psychoactive drug. There are many chemicals called alcohol. Some, such as wood alcohol (methyl alcohol) and rubbing alcohol (isopropyl alcohol) are poisonous even if only taken in small amounts. The one that concerns this book is ethyl alcohol. Only this produces the generally desired effects and is safe to drink in moderate quantities. It is a clear liquid with an astringent taste and very little smell of its own. The smell on the drinker's breath is normally due to other ingredients. Most British beers, lagers, etc. contain 4–7% ethyl alcohol. Spirits contain roughly 40–55% and most wines range from 12–16%. The drug effects of alcohol do not depend upon the specific type of beverage, be it beer, wine or spirits. The important factor is the amount of ethyl alcohol consumed. There is little evidence that any of the other ingredients of alcoholic drinks, known as congeners, have important effects except perhaps on post-intoxication hangovers. A rough guide to the relative alcohol content of different drinks is that half a pint of beer, lager, stout, etc. contains about as much alcohol as either a glass of wine or a single measure of spirits. Some special lagers are roughly twice as strong as ordinary beers. The alcohol content of different drinks is illustrated by Figure 2.1. A single measure of spirits contains much the same amount of alcohol as half a pint of beer. Nevertheless more concentrated drinks (e.g. gin, whisky) have a faster impact upon the drinker's blood alcohol level than do less concentrated drinks (e.g. cider, beer).

Fig. 2.1 *Units of alcohol*

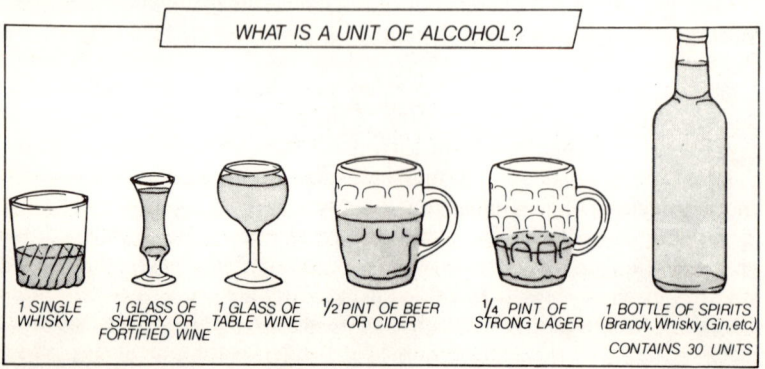

Source: Scottish Health Education Group

Effects

Alcohol is a depressant or a sedative/hypnotic. It slows down all of the activities of the central nervous system. This is contrary to the popular misconception that because people often become more active and feel less inhibited after drinking, it must be a stimulant. Alcohol depresses the general level of activity and in so doing reduces the drinker's inhibitions. It therefore does often create a feeling of relaxation and may provide 'Dutch courage'. One consequence of this paradox is that people who are in fact less able to perform precise tasks while drinking, misguidedly believe that their abilities are enhanced. A commonplace example of this error is the driver who insists that he or she is better able to drive after a couple of drinks.

The effects of alcohol depend upon many factors. Weight, sex, diet and social setting all influence the precise effects of drinking any specific amount of alcohol. Alcohol is passed from the stomach and intestines into the blood stream and is carried throughout the body. It is mainly disposed of through the liver. Large people are less influenced by any given quantity of alcohol than are smaller people. The rate at which alcohol is disposed of by the body does not depend upon the quantity consumed. The more a person drinks the longer will that person be under the influence of alcohol.

Restrained drinking appears to be not only harmless, but is probably beneficial. Alcohol is an effective relaxant and there is some evidence that those who drink in moderation appear to live rather longer than those in the same society who don't drink at all (Kreitman 1982). Even so, excessive drinking does create serious risks:

> 'Alcohol is a potentially addictive drug and if misused a substance that gives pleasure can lead to insidious but finally incapacitating illness. The reasons for alcohol being misused lie not only in the individual but in his society; if the environment is permissive towards excessive drinking then excessive drinking will go unchecked'. (Edwards 1975)

Many definitions of 'problem drinking' or 'alcoholism' have been used. Most definitions of 'alcoholism' contain three elements:

1 Physical dependence on alcohol,
2 Physical damage caused by excessive drinking,
3 Social problems attributed to alcohol misuse.

The traditional concept of drinking problems was based upon the idea that 'alcoholics' were a distinctive and separate group of drinkers. Being 'alcoholic' was viewed as an all-or-nothing condition, rather like being pregnant. In fact, people may experience none or any number of a range of alcohol-related problems, so that it is debatable at which point a person should properly be called an 'alcoholic'. People who do experience drinking problems are a very mixed group. They do not conform to any single stereotype and their alcohol problems are not in themselves a disease, although excessive drinking may well cause secondary physical or mental illness. Many people sometimes experience minor alcohol-related problems, such as hangovers or social disagreements. In addition many of the serious problems caused by alcohol misuse are caused by drunkenness, which is different from physical dependence.

Physical dependence on alcohol usually takes years to develop. As it does, a person needs to drink more to recreate the original effects. Later, if liver damage is caused, this process will be reversed as the body's ability to oxidise alcohol is reduced. Once physical dependence is established symptoms similar to those of barbiturate withdrawal may occur within a few hours if drinking is curtailed. A common symptom of alcohol withdrawal is known as 'the shakes'. These will usually occur the morning after a dependent drinker's blood alcohol level has fallen during sleep.

Withdrawal from alcohol may be accompanied by hallucinations. Sometimes these may be brief, but if the individual has been drinking excessively for many years they are likely to be more severe. Delirium tremens (DTs) are one of the severest and most rare forms of withdrawal from any psychoactive drug. In many users they resemble a bad LSD 'trip', but may last for much longer, sometimes two or three days. During this period the sufferer experiences nightmarish hallucinations. Sometimes, if untreated, people may die undergoing withdrawal from alcohol. Such deaths are usually due to respiratory failure. Fits or alcoholic epilepsy also occur. Fortunately these are rare in Britain and withdrawal ('drying out') can generally be achieved, with appropriate medical care, without undue discomfort in a week or ten days at most. Prolonged heavy drinking may cause brain shrinkage. In its early stages this does not destroy brain cells, but permanent intellectual impairment may ensue if drinking is not curtailed.

Excessive drinking can cause a wide range of physical disabilities. Some of the most widespread and serious of these involve the liver. Reversible fatty liver, hepatitis and irreversible liver cirrhosis are all too common consequences of excessive drinking. At least half of the liver cirrhosis deaths in Britain are attributable to prolonged excessive alcohol consumption. Gastritis (inflamed stomach) and stomach ulcers are common alcohol-related disabilities. These are reversible only in their early stages. Problem drinkers in alcohol treatment units are often deficient in Vitamin B. One consequence of this is impaired memory. Amnesias and confusion may occur, which can be irreversible. Continued excessive drinking may lead to reduced mental capacity, anaemia, acute and chronic pancreatitis, nerve and muscle impairments, heart disease, tuberculosis, emphysema and cancer of the pharynx. Heavy drinking during pregnancy is associated with birth damage. It has been suggested that there is a *foetal alcohol syndrome* of such harm. Fortunately this syndrome appears to be very rare in Britain. In addition evidence suggests that although alcohol consumption is *associated* with birth damage, it might in fact play a far more minor role in causing such harm than other factors such as smoking, diet, maternal age and social class. There is no evidence that the consumption of one or two drinks once or twice a week during pregnancy is harmful (Plant, M. L. 1985).

The misuse of alcohol is associated with numerous social problems. Many of these relate to drunkenness in public or family settings and to motoring offences. Alcohol misuse is a major cause of accidents and is also identified as a cause of inefficiency and absenteeism in employment.

Tobacco

The tobacco plant *Nicotiana tabacum* and its most potent ingredient, nicotine, were named after Jean Nicot, a sixteenth century French ambassador to Portugal. Nicot emphasised what he believed to be the medical merits of this plant whose use was only adopted by Europeans long after it had been indigenous among the peoples of South America. The introduction of tobacco to Europe did not occur unchallenged. King James VI of Scotland and I of England made this comment in 1664: 'Many in this kingdom have had such a continual use of taking this unsavoury smoke, they are not now able to resist the same, no more than an old drunkard can abide to be long sober.' Sadly King James later revised his stance on tobacco once he was alerted to its taxation potential. Tobacco is usually smoked in cigarettes or pipes. It may also be sucked, chewed or sniffed (in the form of snuff). Contrary to Nicot's enthusiasm for its properties, tobacco is now generally accepted to be a major health hazard.

Effects

Tobacco is a stimulant drug but also has some depressant effects. The short-term effects include an increase in heart rate and blood pressure and a fall in skin temperature. Once accustomed to its effects, most smokers are calmed and soothed by tobacco use and some regular users also find inhalation of the smoke greatly satisfying. Those who smoke regularly also cope with amounts of nicotine which would be fatal if taken by a novice. Most smokers smoke every day; some people smoke as many as 100 cigarettes daily, but twenty a day is about average. The principal active ingredient of tobacco is nicotine, which is a highly toxic substance and swallowing even a few drops of the pure alkaloid is fatal. Smoking tobacco only exposes the brain to a relatively small dose of nicotine which is believed to cause most of the effects desired by tobacco users.

There is a vast body of evidence that tobacco is a killer. Smoking is by far the greatest single cause of lung cancer and is associated with cancers of the mouth and respiratory tract. Most of tobacco's long-term effects relate to the bronchopulmonary and cardiovascular systems. Smokers are much more likely than non-smokers to develop coronary heart disease, stomach ulcers and non-malignant diseases of the digestive system. Most of the health problems caused by smoking take several years to develop. Even so, notable short-term effects such as coughs, bronchitis and nausea are quite commonplace even among young smokers. A further threat to health involves the use of so-called 'smokeless tobacco'. A new British factory, the construction of which was assisted by public funds, has been built to manufacture a brand of smokeless tobacco known as 'Skoal Bandits'. These are sachets of tobacco which are chewed or sucked. This unsavoury practice is sometimes referred to as 'snuff dipping'. While the use of such noxious products is new in Britain, it is well established in the United States. A recent report noted that between 8% and 36% of male high school students in the USA are regular users of smokeless tobacco. It has been noted that this form of tobacco use is linked with cancers of the gum and cheek. (Connolly *et al*. 1986, Koop 1986).

Nicotine overdoses are rare, but extremely heavy smoking may cause mild nicotine poisoning which produces headache, shakiness, nausea and possibly diarrhoea. Tobacco smoking by pregnant women is also associated with reduced birth weight. Tobacco smoking certainly often produces psychological dependence, although there are no severe physical withdrawal symptoms. Many smokers clearly wish to give up this habit and studies have shown that this desire is evident even among schoolchildren who have only recently started smoking. Those who do give up smoking tobacco often complain of restlessness and weight gain which can be unpleasant to tolerate. Even so, there are strong motives to justify stopping smoking. The Royal College of Physicians has suggested that each cigarette smoked reduces the smoker's lifespan by 5½ minutes.

Some of the constituents of tars resulting from tobacco cause cancer. Evidence suggests that the carbon monoxide and nicotine in tobacco smoke contribute to heart disease. Most British tobacco produces acidic smoke. This is more easily inhaled than the alkali smoke of cigarettes used in many other countries. Possibly this difference explains why Britain has the highest rate of lung cancer in the world.

Cannabis

Cannabis (marijuana, marihuana, dope, blow, draw, bush, hashish, bhang, kif, ganja, pot, grass, shit, etc.) is derived from the marijuana plant, *cannabis sativa*. This occurs in two varieties, the hemp type and the drug type. These differ in relation to the amounts of the main psychoactive ingredient delta-9-tetrahydrocannabinol (THC) that they contain. The hemp type (used for rope making) contains relatively little of the intoxicating substance, while the drug type contains far greater levels of THC. The marijuana plant occurs in many different forms and may grow as tall as fifteen feet. Cannabis has been used for thousands of years. It was used medically in China 4000 years ago and has been a popular recreational drug since at least 2000 BC in the Indian subcontinent. Subsequently its use spread to the Middle East and North Africa. It was especially attractive in Islamic countries where the use of alcohol is expressly forbidden. Cannabis was adopted by western medical practice during the nineteenth century. Exaggerated claims were made for its value in treating a wide range of ills. In probability much of its 'success' was attributable purely to its placebo value, the psychological effect of taking any pill or potion. The introduction of much more powerful and specifically useful drugs has long since removed the use of cannabis from medical practice. It was used recreationally during the nineteenth century by some western intellectuals such as Gautier and Baudelaire but has only been adopted on a large scale much more recently by young people in industrial countries.

The commonest forms of cannabis available in Britain are:

1 Cannabis resin (hashish) which is the dried caked resin derived from the tops and leaves of the female plant. Cannabis resin usually contains more THC than marijuana and is accordingly more potent. Cannabis resin is available in various forms, some of which superficially resemble dark-coloured chocolate. Others are mustard-yellow and powdery, reddish-brown and crumbly or even greenish-black and sticky.
2 Marijuana, which consists of the flowering and fruiting tops and leaves of the plant. Very often seeds, stems and other parts of the plant are also included.
3 Cannabis oil, a ruddy brown extract from the resin or the plant. It is known by a variety of names, including 'hash oil' or 'liquid hash'. This is the most potent form of cannabis apart from pure THC.

Resin is the form in which cannabis is mainly used in Britain, although marijuana is the form most freely available in the United States. Cannabis is normally smoked, although it may also be chewed or ingested as an ingredient in food or drinks. When smoked, a little cannabis resin is usually mixed with tobacco and rolled into a cigarette called a 'joint'.

Most of the cannabis available illegally in Britain originates from the Indian subcontinent, the Middle East, Africa and the West Indies. Enthusiasts also sometimes grow cannabis plants in Britain, although this is illegal.

Effects

There is little doubt that very often the effects of cannabis depend upon setting, expectations and mood. Many people who experiment with it report little or no effect whatever. It is a depressant drug which, like alcohol, slows reaction time, impairs co-ordination and may induce drowsiness. It is also a mild hallucinogen. The desired short-term reaction is a 'high' or euphoria similar to mild alcohol intoxication. This may be followed by a quieter, passive phase which in turn is followed by sleep. Reddened eyes and increased pulse rate are also commonplace short-term effects. Experienced users report that they achieve the greatest effects by inhaling the smoke and holding it in their lungs. It certainly appears that novices often have to 'learn' how to achieve the desired effects by contact with regular users. Usually cannabis smoking provides only mild and relatively brief effects, but sometimes unpleasant experiences, even hallucinations, do result from use. Cannabis impairs short-term memory and affects ability to perform precise tasks such as driving in much the same way that alcohol does. Larger doses of cannabis certainly sometimes produce unpleasant experiences broadly comparable to those of a bad LSD trip. Such experiences may cause long-term emotional disturbance.

Tolerance may develop very rapidly with cannabis, so that users sometimes need to smoke steadily increased amounts to recapture the original effects of the drug. During a cannabis-induced intoxication or 'high', the pupils of the eyes contract, they do not dilate as popularly believed. THC potentiates with alcohol, amphetamine and tobacco and in consequence, if these substances are used in conjunction their effects are greatly and possibly dangerously magnified. Some cannabis users certainly become psychologically dependent on the drug even though there appear to be few tangible physical withdrawal symptoms. It is certainly not true that cannabis is a 'safe' drug. Derivatives of cannabis accumulate in the tissues of the brain, lungs and the sex glands and prolonged or heavy cannabis use has been found to cause damage in blood cells and in spermatozoa. Animal studies have shown that cannabis use in pregnant mammals increases the incidence of foetal damage and death. Even short-term cannabis use greatly increases the risks of a wide range of lung damage and related disabilities. Cannabis smoking causes far higher levels of such impairment in the short-term than does tobacco smoking. Chronic cannabis use sometimes causes severe psychological impairment. In countries where cannabis has been used for a long time, such as Egypt and Morocco, it has long been regarded, and for good reason, as a major health hazard. There is abundant evidence to support the view that prolonged heavy cannabis use is both physically damaging and likely to lead to loss of motivation, apathy and passivity. This loss of psychological alertness and vigour has been called the 'amotivational syndrome'. To some extent this may be attributable to the ideology and lifestyle of the drug scene rather than the chemistry of cannabis. It is clear that large numbers of cannabis smokers use the drug only intermittently and that they do so without apparent harm. Several major committees of inquiry have concluded that smoking cannabis in moderation is unlikely to cause health damage. Even so, the potential dangers of regular cannabis use are now clear and should be borne in mind.

LSD

This is one of the most dramatic of the psychoactive drugs. LSD 25 (lysergic acid diethylamide) is a drug whose characteristic effect is to distort the way its user sees and senses the world.

DRUGS AND THEIR EFFECTS

Many hallucinogenic drugs (sometimes called 'psychedelics') occur naturally and have long been used in South, Central and North America for recreational purposes or in conjunction with religious ceremonies. These substances include peyote (a cactus) and mescalin (a mushroom).

LSD is by far the most potent of the commonly available hallucinogens. It is a recent product, having first been produced in 1938. Its hallucinogenic effects were noted in 1943 and since then it has been used experimentally in psychiatry (although its use for such purpose is now almost non-existent). The powerful effect of LSD led to its use becoming extremely controversial. It was hailed by some as mind-expanding, a key to self enlightenment or 'instant Nirvana'. Others decried it as unpredictable and mentally destructive. The subjective effects of LSD have been vividly described in Aldous Huxley's *The Doors of Perception*. It is a substance that most users do not take more than once or twice.

Most other hallucinogens such as MDA (methylenedioxy-amphetamine), mescalin, psilocybin, Morning Glory seed and nutmeg are sometimes used but appear to be far less popular than LSD. A variant of MDA is MDMA, better known colloquially as 'Ecstasy'. This is a powerful hallucinogen, the advent of which in the USA caused concern. This is because American law defines drugs as being legal if they are not proscribed by name. This, at the time of writing, is a general problem associated with new synthetic or 'designer' drugs. It is probable that indigenous 'magic mushrooms' are currently used at least as widely as LSD. The latter include Liberty Cap (*Psilocybe semilanceata*) and Fly Agaric (*Aminita muscaria*). This use of such fungi is associated with a variety of toxic effects. The latter include poisoning, hallucinations, nervous tension and disturbed sleep patterns. Fly Agaric is especially dangerous if eaten raw or consumed in large quantities.

Effects

LSD is a very potent drug. Tiny amounts are sufficient to trigger off a 'trip' or experience which may well be psychologically overwhelming and routinely lasts for as long as seven hours. The drug is available in many forms: capsules, microdots or as a liquid. It is usually prepared as a tartrate salt that is water soluble. It is easily carried (smuggled) and is often soaked in sugar or blotting paper. It is usually swallowed but may also be sniffed or injected. The effects normally begin an hour or so after ingestion and reach their peak two to three hours later. The effects do not directly depend on dose and as little as 30 or 40 micrograms are sufficient to produce the desired goal. LSD accentuates and distorts the user's mental and emotional state. There is little doubt that to a large extent the effects depend upon the user's original disposition, company and surroundings and are rather unpredictable. It often causes profound changes in perceptions and mood. These may be extremely pleasant or devastatingly horrifying. Blood pressure often rises and heartbeat may accelerate. Hyperventilation, nausea, weakness and depression may also occur. Occasionally convulsions have been caused by LSD usage. The drug does not cause physical dependence but its potency in changing emotional state does sometimes cause 'bad trips'. These extremely unpleasant experiences may either produce or accentuate extreme mental disorientation and can occur after only a single experimentation.

'Flashbacks' or recurrences of the effects experienced during an LSD trip have been widely reported by users even months after experimentation. Sometimes such flashbacks occur at dangerous or at least embarrassing times. Tolerance to LSD develops rapidly so that the initial effects quickly wane. It has been reported that LSD use during pregnancy causes foetal abnormalities, although this possibility has not been conclusively verified. There certainly have been fatal accidents and suicides attributed to the effects of LSD. Even so, these appear to be extremely rare. While LSD does sometimes produce extremely interesting and enjoyable effects, these cannot be relied upon and users participate in a hazardous game of Russian roulette.

Glues, solvents, paints and aerosols (volatile hydrocarbons)

The Greeks reportedly sniffed gases in conjunction with religious rites. Since the eighteenth century, when nitrous oxide was invented, gases have been used sporadically for recreational purposes and nineteenth century medical students were known to inhale nitrous oxide for pleasure. Modern concern about the sniffing of gases of various types has arisen since the Second World War. During the 1950s glue sniffing was reported in the United States and during the past thirty years has periodically also been noted in Britain and in other countries. Most users appear to be young, of no more than secondary school age, and most do not use these highly toxic and dangerous substances more than once or twice. There is little doubt that the incidence of glue sniffing has sometimes been increased by lurid media coverage. This clearly happened in Canada and some of the recent publicity in Britain has virtually advertised the substances available, their effects and mode of use.

Effects

Volatile hydrocarbons are based upon petroleum and natural gas. They evaporate rapidly at room temperature and if inhaled, enter the bloodstream and are quickly conducted to the brain and liver. In consequence their effects are felt very quickly. They are depressants, slowing respiration, heart rate and speed of mental activity. They are also hallucinogens. The initial effect is an intoxication similar to that of drunkenness. Volatile hydrocarbons are slow to disperse from the body and their smell often lingers long on the breath. The inhalation of all such substances is extremely dangerous and deaths have occurred from asphyxiation and from the uncontrolled and bizarre behaviour that sometimes results. Some deaths have been due to heart damage and others due to suffocation from sniffing out of plastic bags. While the initial effect is often a euphoric 'high', this may be succeeded by disorientation, seizures or loss of consciousness.

Generally the effects of a brief inhalation last only a few minutes. They can be greatly prolonged if the hydrocarbon is concentrated in a bag. Nausea and headaches may ensue which sometimes last several days.

Protracted sniffing has been known to produce a constellation of effects which are reversible if inhalation is ceased. Some of these are thirst, weight loss, nose bleeds, sores on mouth and nose, confusion, forgetfulness, fatigue, depression and paranoia. Reversible or permanent heart, kidney and liver disease may also be caused. Respiratory failure is especially likely to occur if aerosols are sprayed directly into the mouth and inhaled. Rarely, if sniffing is continued over a long period of time, brain damage may also result. Tolerance can be established and some excessive users have certainly become physically as well as psychologically dependent. Extremely bad withdrawal symptoms, comparable to the delirium tremens of severe alcohol withdrawal, have very occasionally been recorded. Glues based upon toluene are toxic; petrol and many paints contain poisonous lead and many aerosols and camping gases also contain poisons. These are all potentially lethal. Many of the long-term effects of volatile hydrocarbons are unclear.

Tranquillisers

1 Benzodiazepines

During the past thirty years tranquillisers have been prescribed in hugely increasing quantities. It has been speculated that in Britain one night's sleep in ten is aided or induced by such drugs and that in the United States this rate could be as high as one in six. The most commonly prescribed tranquillisers are the *benzodiazepines*, commonly marketed under the brand names Mogadon (nitrazepam), Valium (diazepam), Librium (chlordiazepoxide hydrochloride) and Ativan (lorazepam).

The availability of these drugs has led to an increasing level of accidents and misuse and there is little doubt that they are often prescribed unnecessarily and for far too long.

Effects

Valium and Librium are chemically very similar. Both are used to reduce anxiety. Librium was first produced in 1960, Valium was introduced three years later. The former drug was promoted to relieve anxiety, while the second was promoted to cope with 'psychic tension'. The main effect of these drugs is that they relieve anxiety without the marked drowsiness induced by barbiturates. In fact there are a number of serious potential dangers attached to these otherwise useful drugs. Cessation of prolonged regular use may, very rarely, cause severe withdrawal symptoms comparable to those associated with barbiturates. These have involved abdominal and muscle cramps, insomnia, anxiety, depression, convulsions, vomiting and sweating. The overdose 'potential' of benzodiazepines is certainly much lower than that of the barbiturates, but fatalities have been caused by both children and adults swallowing large quantities either accidentally or intentionally. Both Librium and Valium have been shown to cause birth defects if taken during the first forty-two days of pregnancy. Among the abnormalities noted are mental retardation, heart damage, deafness and deformities of joints and intestines. In addition, excessive prescribing of benzodiazepines has caused the following side-effects; drowsiness, depression, altered sexual drive, jaundice, constipation, skin problems and confusion. Such adverse reactions are usually reversible by adjusting the dosage. Sometimes depression resulting from excessive dosage has been interpreted as justifying even higher dosage and some problems arising from the benzodiazepines result from overprescribing. It is essential that the use of these clearly valuable drugs be carefully monitored to prevent patients obtaining or using excessive amounts. In addition, like all tranquillisers, they may be dangerous if mixed with alcohol or other depressant drugs. Such combinations create a risk of both psychological and physical dependence and of overdose.

Lader (1986) has noted:

> '1¼ million of the UK population take benzodiazepines for more than one year although their estimated long-term effectiveness is not established. In addition psychological impairment and neuroradiological changes may be associated with long-term administration . . . Withdrawal symptoms may follow treatment as short as 4–6 weeks'.

2 Other Tranquillisers

Tranquillisers have often been subdivided into 'minor' ones (such as Librium and Valium) and 'major' ones such as the phenothiazines. These terms are misleading since it is not true that 'minor' tranquillisers are necessarily less potent than the 'major' ones. The *phenothiazines* such as Stelazine and Thorazine are mainly used to treat definite psychological disorders such as psychosis or schizophrenia. They are widely used in psychiatry and, at the correct doses, are generally regarded as both useful and safe. They have little 'addictive' potential but if combined with alcohol or other depressant drugs can cause overdoses.

Tricyclic antidepressants such as Tryptizol and Tofranil are widely used to counter depression. They are unlikely to produce dependence but do have a serious overdose potential. Adverse reactions sometimes occur and abrupt withdrawal after regular use may cause nausea and other discomfort.

Barbiturates

Barbiturates are the most widely used drugs that are called 'sedative hypnotics'. They were introduced into medical use in 1903. Over 2000 types of barbiturate have been synthesised and in 1972, 11,688,000 prescriptions for barbiturates were issued in Britain. A vigorous campaign, CURB, has pointed out the dangers of these drugs and has succeeded in achieving a drastic reduction in their use. They have largely, although not completely, been replaced by other, safer drugs. By 1984 the annual number of barbiturate prescriptions had fallen to 1,914,000.

Effects

Barbiturates are central nervous system depressants which slow down or decrease many bodily functions. They have an extremely high overdose potential, especially when mixed with alcohol or other depressants and have often been used as a means of committing suicide. The short-term effects are initially to relieve anxiety and tension. Larger amounts produce intoxication or drowsiness and unconsciousness and coma may result. Like alcohol, barbiturates impair judgement and should never be used when it is necessary to perform skilled tasks, such as driving a car. Continued use may create tolerance. Withdrawal from barbiturates can be both unpleasant and dangerous, involving delirium tremens, occasionally even fatal if not properly supervised. It has been speculated that thousands of people in Britain are physically dependent on barbiturates. These drugs are usually taken orally but they have sometimes been injected by young drugtakers. This practice is extremely dangerous due to non-soluble additives and has caused severe physical disabilities due to infections, blood clots and abscesses.

Mandrax

The active ingredient of Mandrax is methaqualone. It is virtually identical to barbiturates in its effects. Like barbiturates, Mandrax has a very high dependence and overdose potential and the latter is especially dangerous if taken in combination with alcohol or other depressants. Mandrax is reputedly, yet dubiously, believed to have aphrodisiac properties ('randy Mandies'). There is no persuasive evidence to support this belief.

While Mandrax shares many of the properties of barbiturates, dependence is less likely to occur. It has been widely used illegally as a recreational drug.

The opiates – opium, morphine and heroin

The opiates are derived from the juice of the opium poppy (*papaver somniferum*). Their effects have long been known and they have been used for both pleasure and medical purposes for thousands of years. The use of a tincture of opium called laudanum was used for centuries as a cure for diarrhoea and malaria. During the nineteenth century it was used in epidemic proportions in the Fens of East Anglia where poppy-head tea was a common local beverage. Working people in Victorian cities used opium, as did many of the Romantic poets. Its virtues were extolled by Coleridge and de Quincey. The practice of giving opium pills to children continued in Britain until the 1920s (Berridge 1979).

Morphine, a derivative of the opium poppy, was isolated in the mid nineteenth century and has since been available in solution. In this form it was ideal for injection and since the introduction of the hypodermic syringe has widely been used by this means. Heroin (diacetylmorphine) was derived in 1898. Its many colloquial names include 'smack' and 'skag'. Ironically it was produced as the result of a quest for a 'safer', less dependence producing drug than morphine. Subsequently other similar drugs, synthetic or semi-synthetic opiates, have been produced. All have proved to be dependence-producing in their own right. Methadone (Physeptone) is widely prescribed as a preferable alternative for heroin dependents. Dipipanone (Diconal) is another drug that has similar effects to the opiates and is sometimes used as a substitute for heroin.

Effects

The opiates produce euphoria and are painkillers. Heroin is a powerful analgesic and is widely used by doctors to treat pain in cancer and heart attack patients. Morphine is mainly used to relieve pain caused by burns, etc. but is more likely than heroin to raise blood pressure and in consequence is not used for people with high blood pressure. Other opiates or similar drugs are also used as painkillers. Opium is a blackish sticky substance which has long been used as a folk medicine or smoked to produce euphoria for purely recreational purposes.

Morphine and heroin may be injected, but may also be eaten, smoked or sniffed. The immediate effects of heroin and allied drugs are sometimes referred to as 'the rush'. A common way of using heroin is called 'chasing the dragon', which involves heating heroin and inhaling the fumes thus generated. In some ways this is a safer procedure than injecting but may also, if continued, produce dependence. All opiates produce tolerance if used regularly and abrupt cessation of regular use may produce withdrawal symptoms.

The seriousness of opiate withdrawal has been much exaggerated. Sometimes withdrawal after prolonged heavy opiate use is fatal, but such tragic outcomes are very rare in Britain and may well be at least partly attributable to extreme panic rather than to purely physical causes. It is a myth that using opiates a few times *causes* inevitable dependence. Most users only take these substances experimentally and most use does not lead to physical dependence. In addition it is clear that for most users withdrawal symptoms, if they occur at all, are relatively trivial, far less serious than those involved in withdrawal from alcohol, barbiturates or some tranquillisers. Heroin withdrawal symptoms usually occur six to twelve hours after the last dose. They range from minor discomfort, similar to that from a cold, to cramps, nausea, sweating, dilated pupils, diarrhoea, headache and insomnia. Usually withdrawal passes its worst within two to three days and recovery generally takes no more than a week, although it often takes longer for sleep patterns to return to normal.

Withdrawal from methadone is a slower process. It may not begin until a few days after the last dose and often reaches its peak after a further three or four days.

The opiates are themselves not particularly toxic unless taken in great quantities. Much of the damage caused by injecting such drugs is due to lack of hygiene or to impurities mixed with the opiates. Sometimes heroin bought on the black market contains highly dangerous substances which are added to increase the vendor's profit. Unsterile injecting and sharing needles certainly spread hepatitis, syphilis and other diseases and excessive or clumsy injecting sometimes collapses veins. The sharing of infected syringes and needles by intravenous drug users, both in Britain (notably Edinburgh) and elsewhere has been associated with the spread of the AIDS (HIV) virus. Sometimes this very dangerous sharing of equipment occurs in premises known as 'shooting galleries'. It is possible to overdose with opiates, especially if using illegal supplies of uncertain purity. In addition, babies born to women who are using heroin may also be physically dependent and might die unless this condition is detected and treated. Foetuses who have been exposed to the AIDS virus have a high risk of developing AIDS soon after birth.

The 'traditional' array of opiate-like drugs has been augmented by illegally produced synthetic substances popularly known as *designer drugs*. Some of these are extremely potent. At the time of writing these were becoming widely used in the United States but were little used in Britain. The advent of such drugs is ominous not only because of their alleged potency, but also because they do not need to be imported and might therefore be harder to control than conventional opiates.

Amphetamines

The first large-scale manifestation of illegal recreational drug use among British teenagers involved the use of amphetamines, colloquially known as 'speed' or 'uppers'. Amphetamine was first synthesised in 1887 but was not widely used medically until the 1930s. Amphetamines of various types were prescribed on a large scale as slimming pills or to alleviate mild depression. Amphetamines are available in a profusion of forms. They can be categorised into three groups with different but related structures; amphetamine e.g. Benzedrine; dexamphetamine e.g. Dexedrine, and methylamphetamine e.g. Methedrine. Amphetamine is also contained in a wide range of tranquillisers and other drugs such as Drinamyl, Durophet-M and Tranquel. In addition some other drugs such as Ritalin, Filon and Ronyl have broadly similar effects to amphetamine.

The extensive availability of these drugs enabled them to be obtained illegally by young people who used them recreationally on a hitherto unprecedented scale. During the 1960s amphetamines were widely misused (readers may recall the 'black bombers', 'purple hearts' and 'French blues' of the 1960s Mods and Rockers era). Amphetamine misuse reached its peak in Japan where it was estimated that 500,000 people used them non-medically in 1954. During the Vietnam War American soldiers used huge quantities of amphetamine tablets. The scale of misuse of these drugs coincided with growing awareness that a major reason for extensive amphetamine misuse was the huge stocks of these drugs in chemists' shops which could quite easily be stolen for black market purposes. Following the lead of a group of doctors in Ipswich the British medical profession adopted a severe voluntary reduction of amphetamine prescribing. These drugs are still sometimes used for rather unusual conditions such as narcolepsy (uncontrolled fits of sleep) and hyperactivity in children. Since 1969 it has been an offence to possess amphetamines without medical authorisation.

Effects

Amphetamines are stimulants, which produce feelings of energy and confidence. They increase heart rate, blood pressure and the level of blood sugar. The pupils are dilated and appetite is suppressed. The rate of breathing is accelerated and they enable users to remain awake for longer periods. For these reasons they have been used illegally to stay awake at parties, dances and concerts or simply to generate a feeling of euphoria. In many ways the effects of amphetamines resemble those of adrenaline. They act not only on the brain but also on the lungs, heart and other parts of the body. The type and scale of the effects depend largely upon the amounts used. The effects are greatest if amphetamine is injected into a vein, and smallest if taken orally. Larger doses may cause dry mouth, sweating, shakiness, blurred vision and headache. Extremely large quantities may lead to flushing, pallor, changed and possibly irregular heartbeat, loss of co-ordination and sometimes psychotic or irrational behaviour. Excessive amphetamine use has, rarely, led to fatalities due to burst blood vessels in the brain and heart failure.

While with low doses users often feel euphoric, it is easy to experience unpleasant effects at higher levels of use. Aggressive and violent behaviour has been attributed to amphetamine taking. In addition, tolerance develops rapidly with amphetamines. Psychological dependence sometimes develops and although there are no *physical* withdrawal symptoms, withdrawal may cause severe, even suicidal, depression combined with hunger, fatigue and irregular sleep patterns. Amphetamine psychosis, which sometimes ensues from taking large doses of the drug, is usually reversible and fades a few days or weeks after cessation of use.

Pure amphetamine is in the form of yellowish crystals. Most legally produced amphetamines are in pill form, but it is also sometimes available as a liquid (injectable methedrine) or crystalline powder (amphetamine sulphate). Most of the illegally available amphetamine is in the form of amphetamine sulphate. This is usually sniffed but may also be eaten or smoked in a mixture with tobacco. Illegal users ('speed freaks') have injected either liquid amphetamine such as methedrine, or a solution made by adding water to amphetamine sulphate. The impurities sometimes contained in these illicit mixtures, like those sometimes present with injected barbiturates, may cause skin sores, blocked blood vessels or other problems. Prolonged heavy use of amphetamine, especially if it is injected, causes a syndrome of under-nourishment, insomnia and often infection and mental disturbance.

While the effect of moderate doses of amphetamine may be pleasant, it often produces restlessness, anxiety and over-confidence. Amphetamine does not create energy, it simply uses it up, so that use is invariably followed by fatigue, often combined with irregular sleep patterns. This is known as the amphetamine 'crash'.

Few deaths have been directly attributable to amphetamine use, although hepatitis, malnutrition and other infections are commonplace among users and it is possible to overdose with amphetamines.

Angel Dust (PCP)

One of the nastiest and most toxic substances to be widely used recreationally during recent years is 'Angel Dust' (phencyclidine hydrochloride). This substance, also colloquially known as PCP, crystal, super grass, goon, scuffle, peace weed or hog, was first produced as an animal anaesthetic. It has been widely used and misused in the United States for some years and is associated with a great many problems.

Effects
PCP is a hallucinogen and a stimulant. It is available either as 'Angel Dust' in crystalline form, or may easily be dissolved in water. It may be injected, smoked (in cigarettes or 'joints' known as 'dusters'), sniffed or swallowed as a powder, in food or as a beverage. The usual or desired effects of PCP are a 'high' accompanied by a feeling of detachment, dreaminess or pleasant or exciting hallucination. In fact, the effects may be dramatically unpleasant and it is extremely easy to overdose and to produce dangerous consequences. Even when a 'normal' high wears off, depression, panic or psychosis may ensue. Overdosing may cause stupor, unconsciousness, vomiting or convulsions as well as bizarre, even criminally destructive (or self-destructive) behaviour. In America PCP has been the cause of numerous crimes and some horrifying acts of aggression or self-mutilation. There is plenty of evidence to suggest that if this spreads to Britain, as other drug fashions have done, it will

have tragic consequences. The high overdose potential of PCP is a major hazard, which may lead to respiratory failure. Its only 'legitimate use', as an animal tranquilliser, is being curtailed because of its convulsive side-effects, and replaced by safe alternatives.

Cocaine

Cocaine is derived from the coca plant which grows in South America, South East Asia, Africa and the West Indies. Coca has been used for centuries in South America as a cure for a variety of ailments such as rheumatism, and as a stimulant. The Incas regarded coca as not just acceptable but as a divine plant with magical properties. Its use was considered to be a mark of high social status. The coca plant, which grows up to about three feet in height, probably originated in South America. It exists in several cultivated varieties which contain only a small proportion of pure cocaine. Cocaine was not isolated until the mid nineteenth century and is far more powerful and potentially dangerous than the much milder coca with which it has often wrongly been equated.

Effects

Cocaine is a stimulant and as such may be broadly compared with the amphetamines. It is mainly used medically as a local anaesthetic or a pain blocker. Cocaine is a white crystalline powder. When used recreationally it is usually sniffed or smoked and this induces alertness and energy. Cocaine may produce intense euphoria which in turn may make this one of the most psychologically compelling of drugs and psychological dependence may result from continued use. Physical dependence does not appear to develop but withdrawal may be accompanied by severe discomfort which is probably attributable to panic but which can be manifested by physical symptoms. Sherlock Holmes apart, cocaine has never been widely used in Britain. It has been expensive to buy illegally and for this reason was once restricted in availability in both Britain and America and was regarded as a 'chic' exclusive drug. During recent years the supply of cocaine has increased tremendously and its price has fallen, so that it is no longer a 'luxury drug'. Sniffing cocaine is a potentially very dangerous practice which can erode through the septum of the nose. Injecting cocaine, like injecting any drug, may spread hepatitis, AIDS or other forms of infection if equipment is shared. Cocaine may be smoked. The crystals are heated and the resulting fumes are then inhaled. This procedure is called 'freebasing'.

During recent years cocaine misuse has been identified as the fastest growing illegal drug problem in the United States. As prices have fallen cocaine has become far more widely used than ever before. The current type of cocaine, which is commonly smoked, not sniffed, is often called 'crack' or 'rock'. The term 'crack' refers to the noises caused by heating cocaine to produce this drug. It is reportedly far easier to become psychologically dependent upon this form of cocaine than upon the older variety. Freebasing accentuates the risk that use will provoke toxic psychosis.

'Dealers make crack by mixing cocaine with common baking soda and water, creating a paste that is usually at least 75 percent cocaine. The paste hardens and is cut into chips that resemble soap or whitish gravel. A small piece, sometimes called "a quarter rock" produces a 20 to 30 minute high. It is usually smoked in water pipes'. (Newsweek 1986)

The range of substances that are sometimes used to produce a change of consciousness is enormous and perplexing. Devotees of drug experimentation have smoked virtually every product from health-food shops and have combed the woods and hedgerows for magic mushrooms or other mind-expanding vegetation. The preceding descriptions probably cover the major types of psychoactive drugs that are used in Britain. In addition, a profusion of cough mixtures, inhalants, syrups and other drugs are sometimes taken recreationally. Even humble kitchen items such as nutmeg have been used to produce a 'high'. (Such use of nutmeg is a dangerous practice.) Any substance that generates a pleasant feeling may be used excessively or unwisely, regardless of whether or not it produces physical dependence. The chemistry of drugs is important. Some are clearly potentially dangerous, either in the short-term, such as LSD or glues and solvents, or less obvious though equally important longer-term dangers, such as tobacco and cannabis. Some, like alcohol and a wide range of tranquillisers, have positive effects if used sensibly and in moderation but may produce tragic consequences if taken excessively. The effects of a drug depend not only upon its chemistry but upon the user, the purpose for which it is used, its legal and social status and the quantities and frequency of use.

3 Why People Use Drugs

A daunting number of suggestions have been put forward to explain why people use drugs and why some users become dependent upon them. Many of the suggestions are speculative to the extent that they stem from personal experiences and observation of specific drugtakers rather than upon rigorous research. Most theories about the *causes* of drug use or drug dependence rely upon descriptions of the features of *established* drugtakers. There is very little information about the characteristics of these individuals before they become involved with drug use. For this reason there has been frequent confusion between the *causes* of drug use and its apparent *correlates* or even *consequences*.

Most British studies of drug users have been confined to highly selective groups such as students or people in treatment institutions. Even surveys of tobacco smoking and alcohol consumption have been mainly limited either to small samples or to specific geographical areas. The important differences noted between different groups such as heroin dependants in a clinic or cannabis smokers in colleges and universities have been largely responsible for the different causal theories put forward. Virtually every writer on the subject of drug use has ventured some opinion on the likely reasons for such behaviour, be it casual experimentation or physical dependence. Most writers have highlighted ideas that are especially relevant to *their* particular study group of drugtakers, but which may have little relevance to others. While a perplexing number of equally plausible and useful theories co-exist it is apparent that drug use in general is the outcome of interactions between the drug, the personal characteristics of the individual and the environment. Few people would suggest that either drug use in general or drug dependence are caused by any single factor. Drug use certainly stems from many reasons and is the subject of many research interests; for example, biological, social, psychological, historical and economic. It would be unrealistic to conclude that research in any single field has all the answers.

Three general types of theory have been suggested. These are constitutional, individual and environmental.

Constitutional (or biological) approaches

These are concerned with either biological predispositions or with the relationship between a drug and the body.

It has been suggested that depressant drugs such as alcohol, barbiturates or tranquillisers might appeal to those in need of relaxation while stimulants, such as cocaine and amphetamines, might appeal to extroverts who are predisposed to hyperactivity. Animal research has shown that sometimes there does exist a genetic predisposition to use specific drugs. There is a growing body of evidence that inherited factors can predispose some people to develop alcohol-related problems. Such factors interact with availability, social context and other important influences on drug use.

During recent years considerable interest and excitement has been aroused by the discovery that the body produces opiate-like substances. It has been known for over twenty years that the human brain has specific receptors for opiates. These receptors, in addition to responding to externally produced opiates such as morphine and heroin, respond to a group of internally produced *peptides*. Some of these substances, called *endorphines* (literally 'the body's own morphine') closely resemble opiates. The receptors excited by such substances are concentrated in the pathways of the brain that are concerned with the perception of pain. In consequence it is an important and intriguing possibility that the development of opiate dependence by some people, or even the general use of certain drugs, may be explained by the ability of some substances to modify the perception of profound experiences such as pleasure and pain.

Individual approaches

Individual approaches are largely concerned with either unusual personality traits (in the cases of drug dependent individuals) or far more general factors such as extroversion which may explain willingness to experiment with cannabis or to indulge in other forms of drug use.

Personality characteristics

It is a commonplace belief that drug dependence is at least partly attributable to personality peculiarities. Many studies have supported this conclusion. Even so the evidence to sustain this view is confusing, to say the least, because it is based upon various groups of drugtakers compared with various 'others'. It does appear that opiate users are probably no more extroverted than normal people, but that they are more neurotic. Even so, this is not a universal conclusion. Some institutionalised drugtakers have been noted to exhibit higher than average 'hostility scores', but are not unique in so doing.

It has been widely noted that most drug use is not evidently attributable to personality abnormalities. The latter may be related to severe drug problems and are often noted among those in clinical settings. Even so it does not appear that there is any unique 'alcohol dependent', 'heroin dependent' or other type of drug dependent personality. In more general terms it has been noted that if any kind of drug is widely acceptable, as is alcohol, then there is no reason at all why users should have unusual personalities.

Intelligence

Evidence shows that drugtakers are of average or above average intelligence. This conclusion is supported by studies of drugtakers in treatment, educational and penal institutions and in the general population. It is clear that drugtakers vary a great deal in many respects, and there is little support for the view that drug use is caused in many cases by lack of intelligence.

General psychiatric state

It is evident that drug dependants in treatment institutions are often psychiatrically disturbed. Sometimes this could result from drug misuse, but there is also evidence that sometimes individuals displayed signs of disturbance before becoming drugtakers. Case history data are often cited to support the view that drugtaking satisfies a variety of psychological needs and that sometimes at least drug dependence is secondary to some clearly defined psychiatric illness. Different studies vary a great deal. Some have concluded that most institutionalised drug users had histories of prior mental illness. Others have concluded that most had not. It is clearly possible that both psychiatric disturbance and drugtaking may be caused by some other factor. It cannot necessarily be assumed that they invariably lead to each other.

Sex

Males appear far more likely than females either to use psychoactive drugs (tranquillisers and depressants excepted) or to be heavy users or dependent upon such substances. These differences are described in more detail in Chapters 4 and 5. There may be many explanations of why males are particularly likely to use drugs. Biological or personality differences between the sexes may predispose males to be drugtakers: males are more aggressive. Certainly social pressures have traditionally inhibited females even from using legal and socially approved drugs such as alcohol and tobacco (although these inhibitions are waning; some evidence suggests that young women may now be more likely to smoke than young men).

Age

Most illegal drug users are young, as are most of those who experience alcohol-related problems such as drunkenness. There has been much speculation about whether or not age does affect drug dependence. It is probable that youthful anxieties and sexual uncertainties may sometimes encourage the use of drugs that enhance relaxation. Also the menopause in women, and old age in general, may often generate pressures that make drug use attractive. On the other hand, if drug use is attributable, as is sometimes suggested, to a personality predisposition there is no reason why it should be especially prevalent among certain age groups.

Drug use as self-medication

Most of the drugs that are used or misused have definite, and usually relaxing, effects. Sometimes such drugs are prescribed by doctors for precisely this reason. It is a possibility that people who have high anxiety levels or other strong psychological needs use drugs specifically to adjust their 'unsatisfactory' mental states to a more acceptable condition. Many drug users certainly report that they do use drugs 'to get high', 'to feel relaxed', 'for the experience'. Often this motivation appears to be quite casual. Individuals who are drug dependent also frequently account for their reliance upon drugs in similar terms. 'I use drugs to stop being depressed.'

It is difficult to assess how truthful or perceptive such accounts are. Precise motivations for complex acts are hard to pin down with accuracy. The main problem is that one cannot guess what would have become of an individual if drugs had not been used. That depression and anxiety are commonplace features among drug dependent people is not reason enough to conclude that drug use was adopted as a calculated means of countering such conditions.

Hedonism

Drugs can be fun. They offer an accessible and often reliable means of obtaining enjoyable experiences. Anyone who doubts this should consider the fact that most adult humans use drugs and appear to accept uncritically the view that such use is valuable. Accounts by drugtakers make it very evident that many, if not most, use drugs because they consider their use if not practically useful, at least pleasant. Psychoactive drugs by definition alter the user's mental state, either slowing, speeding or distorting perceptions. Many autobiographical accounts of drug use have described and emphasised the important appeal of these pleasant effects. Most drug use is indulged in as a facet of other leisure pursuits which are themselves widely considered a source of pleasure.

A basic human need?

As noted above, psychoactive drug use is virtually universal in some form or other. It has been suggested that this may be so because there is a basic human need to experience an altered state of consciousness. This is compatible with the fact that most people use drugs and most people are clearly not psychologically disturbed. Altered states of consciousness are attainable in other ways. Meditation, music or mountaineering are among countless alternatives to drug use. This is really a philosophical theory but does merit consideration in face of the willingness of such huge numbers of people to use drugs in whatever way and for whatever effect.

Curiosity

Numerous studies of drug use in social settings report that curiosity is often stated to be the reason for initial drug use. This is as true of alcohol and tobacco as it is of cannabis, LSD, glues, cocaine or opiates. This view, by the drugtakers themselves, may be partisan. Even if curiosity does often account for *initial* drug use, it does not explain why some users become dependent while others do not.

Self destruction/risk taking

The obvious dangers of unwise or excessive drug use have led to speculation that sometimes drugtaking is prompted by self destructive impulses. Alcohol dependence, for example, has been called 'chronic suicide'. This theory is compatible with the fact that many institutionalised drugtakers appear to have poor self-images and sometimes have quite strong feelings of hostility directed at themselves. It is also consistent with the fact that some drugtakers, for whatever reasons, do take overdoses of psychoactive substances. Another theory resulting from the obvious potential dangers of some types of drug use is that it is a form of risk taking. There is little clear evidence that drugtakers in general are particularly predisposed to take risks. Even so, it does appear that some individuals probably choose drugs which produce effects compatible with their personalities or emotional needs.

Resolution of personal problems

Clinical studies indicate that many drug dependent people have serious personal problems. In addition, youthful illegal drug use is often a symbolic gesture of defiance against parental or authority values. It is also possible that adopting the lifestyles of the drugtaker (or the public bar 'regular') provides some people with friendship and social support. There is little doubt that strong social pressures exist, encouraging individuals to conform to certain patterns of drug use as part of more general lifestyles. Even so it remains difficult in individual cases to deduce whether drug use is attributable to prior poor social relationships or exactly what the appeal of drug involvement really is.

Environmental approaches

Environmental approaches relate rates of drugtaking to wider social or cultural factors. Many studies have examined the life experiences of drugtakers, emphasising issues such as broken homes, delinquency, educational or occupational disadvantages. It has also been suggested that social changes or deprivation sometimes precipitate or foster certain types of drug use. The following section examines some of these environmental factors.

Family disturbance

Much attention has been focused on the family background of drugtakers, especially of drug dependent individuals in treatment institutions. Many studies of such clinic populations have noted that a high proportion have come from abnormal or disturbed homes and that excessive drug use or drug dependence does sometimes appear to have been contributed to by family problems of some sort.

The suggested link between drug misuse and parental separation or other family disruptions becomes far less clear-cut when drugtakers are compared with other people. There is no clear evidence that drugtakers *do* differ in this respect from non-drugtakers. In addition, surveys provide abundant evidence that the majority of casual or experimental drug users do not originate from disturbed homes.

There is clear evidence that many institutionalised drug dependants (including problem drinkers) report having parents who were themselves alcohol or drug misusers or who were otherwise unhappy or disturbed. It is widely noted that institutionalised drug dependants often come from 'loveless homes' or have been 'excessively protected'. An evident result of this appears to be the limited abilities of some of these individuals to form satisfactory relationships or to communicate with other people. There is little doubt that very often one generation will imitate the drug use of their predecessors. Parents who use drugs excessively may well produce children who do the same, even if they do so with substances of which their parents strongly disapprove, such as cannabis and heroin.

Unemployment, education and work problems

There is abundant and convincing evidence that many institutionalised young drugtakers exhibit signs of educational disturbance, particularly truancy. In addition many 'drop out' of further or higher education or have had very poor employment records and considerable experience of unemployment. Growing evidence suggests that illegal drug use in the United Kingdom is *associated* with unemployment. In contrast tobacco use has declined as unemployment has risen and alcohol use is not as clearly connected to unemployment, but is also markedly influenced by people's spending powers. Young unemployed people do appear to be particularly likely to use illegal drugs, but the relationship between drugs and unemployment is complex and requires further research. It is apparent that *some* drugtakers have experienced education difficulties *before* their involvement with drugs. Some drug dependent people certainly experience both educational and work difficulties either because of their excessive drug use or possibly as yet another symptom of a more general malaise.

Social class

Drugtaking and drug dependence occur at all social levels. Illegal drug use in America has often been connected with severe social deprivation, for example among poor urban ghetto dwellers. A similar picture has developed in some deprived areas of Britain. Even so, drug dependants in general, including those dependent upon either alcohol or opiates, are drawn from all social classes. As described in Chapter 6 there is evidence that some high status professions have very high rates of alcohol-related problems.

The literature on drugtaking in different social settings indicates that various forms of drug use occur among young people from all types of social class backgrounds. The youthfulness of many drugtakers implies that few will have attained their final occupational levels. Even so many surveys have shown that illegal drug use is quite commonplace at an experimental level among students (who are predominantly from non-manual backgrounds). It does seem that social class influences modes or fashions of drug use. This is clearly so not only in relation to illegal drugs but also in relation to alcohol and tobacco use. It has been suggested that individuals from working class backgrounds are especially likely to be heavy or excessive users of a wide range of drugs. Those from middle class families are generally more restrained and selective.

Peer pressure

One of the most commonly given reasons for initial drug use is peer pressure and a very large number of studies support this view. These range from surveys of teenage drinking and smoking to studies of how people first became cannabis smokers or users of other illegal drugs. It is clear from all this evidence that most people begin using drugs, if not from curiosity, then from peer pressure and probably from a combination of both. In addition it is evident that most youthful drugtakers are introduced to drug use by friends of their own age and background. This conclusion appears to be as applicable to heroin injectors as to cannabis smokers. The phenomenon of 'proselytising' or seeking to convert others to drug use was widely discussed in relation to youthful heroin use during the 1960s. Some young people appear to be especially likely to be subject to social pressures to indulge in drug use. These include the unemployed, people whose jobs foster drinking or students and others living away from their parental homes in flats, bedsitters or halls of residence. All are likely to be exposed to, if not influenced by, the fashions and enthusiasms of their peers. Sometimes this pressure will generate strong social endorsement for using cannabis, LSD or heroin.

There is plentiful evidence to support the view that peer pressure is often a potent reason for beginning or continuing drug use. This conclusion rests largely upon self-reporting by drug users who may be reluctant to concede that their use was motivated by any 'abnormal' causes. It is also possible that disturbed or 'impressionable' individuals may be particularly susceptible to peer pressure. This is consistent with the frequently expressed criticism that drug use is sometimes due to 'falling into bad company'. The fact is that from the drug user's point of view the company is often very good. It is clear that people will normally only be influenced by those whom they regard as acceptable, if not exemplars, people whom they like and wish to be accepted by.

It is important to note that most young people do appear to be 'converted' to drugtaking by others of their own age on a friendly and obliging basis. *There is very little evidence to support the view, beloved of certain tabloid newspapers, that innocent children are lured on to the rocks of addiction by commercially motivated traffickers or pushers lurking outside the nursery.*

Ideology

Some types of drug use are much more widely accepted and indulged in than others. Alcohol and tobacco are widely viewed as symbols of maturity and sociability. Medically prescribed tranquillisers or sleeping tablets are not seen in this way, and their use is much less discussed or publicly paraded. The illegal drugs and various substances used by young people are often regarded as being indicative of protest about or rejection of certain conventional attitudes and values. There is a clear relationship between political and religious ideology and the use of illegal drugs. Self-reports by young drugtakers, especially those deeply involved with drug use, showed that during the 1960s and 1970s most regarded themselves as radical politically and as not sharing their parents' religious views. It could be that the illegal nature of such drug use deters people with conventional, orthodox beliefs. It certainly seems that strong religious views may 'insulate' young people from experimenting with illegal drugs. During the 1960s drug use, especially that of cannabis and LSD, was widely linked with the emergence of a distinctive 'teenage culture' associated in the public mind with permissiveness and hedonism. 'Turn on, tune in, drop out' and other slogans clearly linked illicit drug use with the hippy movement and with a variety of 'new' religious cults, often imported indirectly from the Orient via California. Religion certainly appears to influence alcohol use and is often a reason why people choose not to drink at all. This applies not only to Islamic countries but also to certain Scottish islands and to large areas of the United States.

Delinquency

Many institutionalised drug dependants had criminal records preceding their drug use. This is true of some institutionalised problem drinkers as well as those misusing illegal drugs. As noted above, any type of unusual or anti-social behaviour may predispose those indulging in it to break other social conventions. For this reason people who were previously criminal may be more prepared to begin using illegal drugs than would others. In addition some of the factors which foster illegal drug use may be the same as those promoting other types of crime. In spite of this, the overwhelming majority of those using illegal drugs are not otherwise delinquent.

Occupation

Those in medical, nursing and allied occupations have long been known to be highly at risk of becoming drug dependent. Until the post-war upsurge of youthful heroin use, virtually the only people known to be dependent on opiates in Britain were those in professions who had ready access (usually to morphine) or individuals who had become drug dependent during the course of medical treatment. Doctors have widely been reported to have high rates of alcohol problems. This conclusion was reached by liver cirrhosis rates for the early 1970s. As noted on p98 this may no longer be true. It is important to note that the medical profession is relatively well informed about the effects of drugs. As noted elsewhere in this book, this further weakens the view that drug problems often arise from lack of knowledge. Some occupations certainly expose people to distinctive social pressures and other stresses. Insecure school-leavers starting work or becoming students are often willing to be swayed by encouragement to use drugs which they might have avoided when living with their parents. As noted above, the lack of a job might be a very potent reason for illegal drug use.

Availability

To a large extent, as noted in Chapter 1, specific drugs are used because they are available. Most social groups use whatever substances they have ready access to. The extent of alcohol and tobacco use has widely been attributed to their high levels of availability. In addition there is abundant evidence that the consumption of any drug, be it heroin or alcohol, is influenced by its price compared with that of alternatives.

The upsurge of illegal drug use during the 1960s has been attributed in large measure to the introduction of new types of drugs, either because they had just been invented or because they were being imported from other countries. The fashion for using amphetamines recreationally was certainly encouraged by the vast quantities of these drugs available either through thefts or through prescription. In addition the upsurge in youthful heroin use in the 1960s and 1970s was clearly exacerbated by over-casual prescribing so that 'spare' supplies could be passed on to others eager to experiment. Studies of various groups of drugtakers show that whatever their previous characteristics and inclinations, the availability of drugs in conducive surroundings was an important reason for initial use. The National Health Service is a major supplier of drugs in Britain. Prescribed drugs have certainly sometimes been re-sold, stolen or just left around for others to take. Some of those receiving prescribed drugs have accidentally become 'therapeutically dependent' upon opiates, barbiturates, tranquillisers and other substances. It is evident that even drugs which are considered to be relatively 'safe', such as Ativan, Librium and Valium, will be misused, for example to overdose, provided that they are available in sufficient quantities.

Contact with drugtakers and the opportunity, if so motivated, to use drugs appear to be commonplace conditions for use. Availability is important and appears to influence patterns of drug use in a given area at a given time. Many youthful drugtakers, particularly those in treatment institutions, appear to be willing to use whatever substances are available. Not all individuals are so catholic in their drug tastes. Even so it has often been noted that when, for any reason, large amounts of any drug are available at a reasonable price from whatever source, their use and misuse will invariably increase. Availability does not explain why only some people use drugs or experience drug-related harm. Even so the famous 'Ipswich Experiment', when doctors voluntarily curtailed amphetamine prescribing, proved beyond doubt that controlling the supply of drugs may sometimes drastically reduce their misuse. Such restrictions will, of course, only work if the demand for such drugs is comparatively low and if no effective unofficial or illegal alternative sources of supply exist. The classic western example of an attempt to control the availability of a drug was Prohibition in the United States, 1920–33. During this period, while 'conventional' alcohol-related problems, such as liver cirrhosis, declined enormously, others emerged in the form of bootlegging and gangsterism. Even in Britain today it is clear that proscribing a wide range of drug use requires considerable Customs, police, court and penal resources. In addition, restricting the legitimate supply of any drug creates the risk that illicit supplies may be sought instead. These may be poorly manufactured, adulterated or impure. In addition infringements upon civil liberties and imposing harsh penalties to restrict the use of certain drugs may cause more harm than the drugs themselves would otherwise do.

Historical reasons

There has been considerable discussion about why certain types of drug use, especially recreational drug use by young people, blossomed when it did. Very often the explanations are clear cut. The introduction of tobacco to Britain by Sir Walter Raleigh and the production of new drugs by the pharmaceutical industry clearly facilitated hitherto undreamed of modes of drug use. The emergence of a distinctive youthful drug culture during the 1950s and 1960s probably occurred for a variety of reasons, many of which remain only partly understood.

It has been noted that even during the 1940s and earlier, a certain amount of drug trafficking was carried on by seamen. The use of cannabis received a certain amount of encouragement by North American musicians. Even so, there is little to suggest that either of these influences went much beyond the dockyard gates or the fringes of the avant-garde. The influx of West Indian and Asian Commonwealth immigrants during the 1950s certainly introduced for the first time to Britain fairly large numbers of people used to smoking cannabis. Some of these immigrants certainly continued their cannabis smoking, but there is little evidence to suggest that they actively influenced the host community to participate in this. While immigrant cannabis use was probably fairly self-contained, it may have contributed to the general spread of the recreational use of 'new' types of drug. It is also probable that, like many other fashions from wearing jeans to break dancing, certain type of drug use were adopted due to American influence.

The whole lifestyle of young adults changed during the 1960s. Rock music, 'permissiveness' and 'hippy culture' arrived and support was given to drug use by cult figures such as the new generation of millionaire rock superstars. During this period, 'youth culture' became established with a heavy emphasis on rebellion against established conventional values and practices. Drugs were portrayed by the media as forbidden fruit – dangerous yet exciting. In addition the significance of drugs was enhanced by their links with other popular youthful preoccupations, music and a search for new experience. Often the drugs used complemented the type of music or literature preferred. Amphetamines accompanied strident disco rhythms and helped dancers to stay awake. Cannabis soothed the strains of softer sounds and LSD use was consistent with reading *Lord of the Rings* or listening to Pink Floyd. The music of the period was also explicitly drug oriented and further fostered the integration of drug use with the general youth culture. Since the advent of the recession a far less colourful and romantic set of styles have been apparent. These include punk rock, glues and heroin.

It has been suggested that often illegal drug use is *caused* by the activities of drug traffickers or dealers. In fact, as noted elsewhere in this book, most studies have concluded that initial drug use is largely attributable to encouragement by friends and close associates. The *direct* influence of commercially motivated suppliers has almost certainly been over-emphasised. In more general terms there is a great deal of evidence supporting the view that youthful drug use largely spread in a friendly and hospitable way and reflected much wider social changes. Even so drug use is fostered both by demand and supply and, as noted by Freemantle (1985), the international drug trade is a massive and relentlessly expanding industry. There is no doubt that the network of drug distributers is now developed in the United Kingdom as never before.

The increase in officially recorded drug dependence during the 1960s may have been a logical corollary of the growing acceptance of all forms of drug use. Because relatively large numbers of people were prepared to experiment with substances such as cannabis and LSD, a minority may have been encouraged to use opiates. Even so, such a conclusion is by no means certain and the great majority of illegal drug users appear to confine themselves to casual experimentation.

The media certainly publicised and exaggerated the significance of drug use and often dramatised the drugtaking way of life. Possibly parental control weakened. Certainly many young people were better educated and more socially and economically independent than their parents had been at the same age.

Sociological theories

Several sociological theories have been applied to the post-war spread of drugtaking in Britain. Probably the most important views are that drug use reflected an increase in *alienation* or *anomie*. Such theories attributed youthful drug use to the fact that recent social changes had created new pressures, such as competition for jobs and education, with which some individuals could not cope. In consequence those not finding their needs met by the mainstream of society simply opted out. They turned instead for support to an 'alternative' lifestyle, namely the drug scene. This provided status and companionship without the same demands as the mundane, workaday world. Instead of having to accept the constraints of 'straight' society, with its long-term planning and deferment of gratification, the drug scene permitted instant enjoyment. Thus the lifestyle associated with drugtaking was identified as a distinctive sub-culture. This, because of its free and easy values, permitted people to 'do their own thing' and became a haven for individuals who, for whatever reasons, could not or would not fit into the rat-race of the broader society. This view certainly makes some sense of deep involvement with drugtaking. It is also consistent with the fact that many drug dependent people do have psychological problems or are socially deprived. In particular this approach has the merit of linking drug use with the structure of society. Even so this theory does not, in itself, explain why youthful drug use blossomed when it did, since presumably comparable social pressure has existed during earlier historical periods.

Another sociological view is that once a 'deviant' behaviour, such as drugtaking, becomes evident society attempts to control it and inadvertently makes it worse. The logic of this theory is that as drugtaking is labelled and legislated against, those who indulge in it become more secretive and more cut off from the rest of society. Their deviance is 'amplified'. In consequence the social controls against this 'growing' problem are increased which, in turn, forces the deviants further into isolation and so on. This view provides a useful insight into the possible effects of identifying and attempting to curb a newly defined social problem. There is much truth in this view and some illegal drugtakers certainly appear to enjoy the drama conferred upon their activities by legislation and by their competition against those who enforce it.

As this chapter has described, many plausible theories have been put forward to explain why people use drugs and why some become dependent upon them. Each of these theories is consistent with the characteristics of some drugtakers. Even so it is clear that no single theory can account for all types of drug use. Drugtaking and drug dependence appear to be influenced by a great number of factors, constitutional, individual and environmental. Probably different reasons account for different types of drug use. The casual or experimental use of drugs such as alcohol, tobacco or cannabis is probably largely due to social pressures combined with availability. Deep involvement with, or dependence upon, drugs may well be attributable to much more profound factors such as social deprivation or psychological disturbance. In addition other factors may account for why some people remain dependent while others do not.

4 Drugs and the Law

The growth of present controls

Concern about the misuse of drugs is not a new phenomenon. Even so, the twentieth century has witnessed an unprecedented proliferation of the types of drugs available and the emergence of a distinctive youthful drug-using sub-culture. The sale and public consumption of alcohol and tobacco have long been restricted by licensing laws. In addition, the use of opium has been identified as a social problem long before the present. This chapter outlines the development of the current legal measures intended to control the recreational or non-medical use of the 'newer' drugs, such as cannabis, LSD and heroin. In addition, the legal controls relating to alcohol, tobacco and prescribed drugs are outlined.

Illegal drugs

It should be remembered that before Britain attempted to curb opiate use it was once the major trader of such drugs. Between 1839–1856 the Royal Navy used to force the opium trade upon the Chinese in spite of clear awareness of the harm caused by the use of this drug. In 1916 measures were introduced to control the trafficking of cocaine, mainly by prostitutes and servicemen. The *Defence of the Realm Act* (1916) was strengthened by the *Dangerous Drugs Act* (1920) which extended controls to cover all drugs dealt with by the First International Opium Convention, 1912. Between the two world wars drug misuse appeared to decline, except for limited opium trafficking.

In 1924 the Rolleston Committee was convened to examine the British approach to the whole problem of drug dependence. This Committee reported in 1926 and its report established the so-called *British System* of managing drug dependence. The Rolleston Committee interpreted the existing drug legislation to mean that individuals who were drug dependent were sick, and therefore constituted a purely medical problem. In fact the Committee concluded that it was reasonable to provide drug dependants with regular and controlled supplies of drugs as such a policy permitted drug dependants thereby to maintain reasonably 'normal' lives. Doctors who abused this system were liable to have their freedom of prescribing restricted. Until after the Second World War this system was only required to cope with a relatively small number of 'therapeutic addicts', mainly middle-aged people who had become drug dependent as a result of medical treatment or who, like doctors, nurses and allied workers, had become dependent because of the availability of drugs in connection with their work. Between 1935 and 1955 the number of such dependent individuals recorded by the Home Office declined from 700 to fewer than 400.

During the 1950s cannabis smoking began to spread in Britain. At the same time a new type of drug dependant became evident. Unlike the traditional 'therapeutic addict', these new dependants were mainly young and used heroin rather than morphine. Most significantly, they actively encouraged others to adopt their modes of drug use and appeared, very often, to be afflicted with a variety of social and psychological problems and to have adopted a far from 'normal' lifestyle. The arrival upon the scene of these young 'proselytising junkies' reflected a pattern already evident in America and the prospect of a drug problem of North American proportions caused great concern.

In 1958 the Brain Committee was set up to review the situation. Their report in 1961 narrowly preceded a Home Office statement which depicted a major rise in officially recorded heroin dependence. In the face of a deteriorating situation the Brain Committee was reconvened, and in 1965 produced a second report which conceded that there was an alarming increase in drug misuse. During 1961 Britain ratified the Single Convention, an international treaty which bound consenting nations to control the use of a wide range of psychoactive drugs, including cannabis. During 1964 the *Dangerous Drugs (Prevention of Misuse) Act* was passed to give the police greater powers in relation to drug control. The coverage of this Act was extended in 1966 to include LSD, mescalin and DMT. In 1964 the *Dangerous Drugs (No. 2) Regulations* were added to the statute book, as was the *Dangerous Drugs Act* one year later. These pieces of legislation implemented Britain's obligations under the Single Convention. They covered raw opium, coca leaves, poppy straw and cannabis, as well as the derivatives of these raw substances. The police were given controversial powers to search premises if they received sworn evidence that an offence against these regulations was being committed.

In 1965 the Brain Committee recommended that the legitimate supply of heroin should be drastically curtailed. This suggestion was prompted by the fact that some doctors had clearly been over-prescribing and surpluses of heroin thus acquired had been passed on to other non-registered users. The 1967 *Dangerous Drugs Act* implemented this restriction by limiting the number of doctors who could prescribe heroin to a few at specific clinics (see list of addresses in Appendix 1). General practitioners were no longer allowed to prescribe opiates for drug dependence. (They could continue to prescribe such drugs as painkillers, of course.) The treatment centres which opened during 1968 heralded a new era of restricted heroin prescription. At the same time they increased the demand for, and probably the supply of, heroin from illicit sources; initially from China, and more recently from the Middle East and from Afghanistan and Pakistan.

In 1968 the controversial Wootton Report recommended that the penalties for possession and sale of cannabis be reduced. Many of the recommendations of this Report were not enacted, although the penalties for possessing cannabis were reduced. This was introduced by the *Misuse of Drugs Act* (1971) which forms the basis of the United Kingdom's current drug control laws. The Act came fully into force on 1 July 1973 and replaced the legislation of 1964, 1965 and 1967. The Act divided proscribed drugs into three categories according to their harmfulness and specified different maximum penalties for possession, production or sale of drugs in each of these three categories:

Class A Includes opium, heroin, methadone, morphine, pethidine, cannabinol (except when contained in cannabis or cannabis resin), cocaine, injectable amphetamines, LSD, mescalin and psilocybin.

Class B Includes cannabis and cannabis resin, codeine, pholcodine, amphetamines (Methedrine, Benzedrine, Drinamyl, Dexedrine), medium and long-acting barbiturates.

Class C Includes methaqualone (Mandrax) and certain amphetamines (bezphetamine, chlorphentermine, mephentermine and six others all of which are considered less dangerous or potent).

The 1971 Act also enables the Home Secretary to prevent doctors from over-prescribing controlled drugs and to bring new substances under control as the need emerges. In 1977 the definition of 'cannabis' was widened from the flowering and fruiting tops to cover the whole plant, except mature stalk and seed already separated from it. In 1979 'Angel Dust' (PCP) was made an illegal Class A drug. The *Misuse of Drugs Act 1971 (Modification) Order* (1985) added glutethimide, lefetamine and pentazocine to Class B. In addition the same order added 33 tranquillisers of the benzodiazepine group including diazepam, four sedatives and two suppressants to Class C with effect from April 1st 1986.

The maximum penalties permitted by the *Misuse of Drugs Act* (1971) and the *Controlled Drugs Penalties Act* (1985) are summarised in Table 4.1.

In Scotland existing legislation has been used to convict shopkeepers of supplying young people with 'glue-sniffing kits'. The *Intoxicating Substances (Supply) Act* (1985) made it an offence in England, Wales and Northern Ireland to knowingly supply directly or indirectly people under the age of

Table 4.1 Misuse of Drugs Act (1971) offences and maximum penalties

Offence	Mode of prosecution	Class A drug	Class B drug	Class C drug	General
Production or being concerned in the production of a controlled drug.	(a) Summary (b) On Indictment	6 months or £2,000 or both. Life imprisonment or a fine, or both.	6 months or £2,000 or both. Life imprisonment or fine, or both.	3 months or £500 or both. 5 years or a fine, or both.	
Supplying or offering to supply a controlled drug or being concerned in the doing of either activity by another.	(a) Summary (b) On Indictment	6 months or £2,000 or both. Life imprisonment or a fine, or both.	6 months or £2,000 or both. 14 years or a fine, or both.	3 months or £500 or both. 5 years or a fine, or both.	
Having possession of a controlled drug.	(a) Summary (b) On Indictment	6 months or £2,000 or both. 7 years or a fine, or both.	3 months or £500 or both. 5 years or a fine, or both.	3 months or £200 or both. 2 years or a fine, or both.	
Having possession of a controlled drug with intent to supply it to another.	(a) Summary (b) On Indictment	6 months or £2,000 or both. Life imprisonment or a fine, or both.	6 months or £2,000 or both. 14 years or a fine, or both.	3 months or £500 or both. 5 years or a fine, or both.	

Cultivation of cannabis plant.	(a) Summary (b) On Indictment	—	—	— 6 months or £2,000 or both. 14 years or a fine, or both.
Being the occupier or concerned in the management of premises and permitting or suffering certain activities to take place there.	(a) Summary (b) On Indictment	6 months or £2,000 or both. 14 years or a fine, or both.	6 months or £2,000 or both. 14 years or a fine, or both.	3 months or £500 or both. 5 years or a fine, or both.
Offences relating to opium.	(a) Summary (b) On Indictment	—	—	— 6 months or £2,000 or both. 14 years or a fine, or both.
	(a) Summary (b) On Indictment	—	—	— 6 months or £2,000 or both. 2 years or a fine, or both.
Contravention of direction prohibiting practitioner, etc, from possessing, supplying, etc. controlled drugs.	(a) Summary (b) On Indictment	6 months or £2,000 or both. 14 years or a fine, or both.	6 months or £2,000 or both. 14 years or a fine, or both.	3 months or £500 or both. 5 years or a fine, or both.

Table 4.1 *continued*

Offence	Mode of prosecution	Class A drug	Class B drug	Class C drug	General
Contravention of direction prohibiting practitioner, etc. from prescribing, supplying, etc. controlled drugs	(a) Summary (b) On Indictment	6 months or £2,000 or both. 14 years or a fine, or both.	6 months or £2,000 or both. 14 years or a fine, or both.	3 months or £500 or both. 5 years or a fine, or both.	
Failure to comply with notice requiring information relating to prescribing, supply, etc. of drugs.	Summary	—	—	—	£400
Giving false information in purported compliance with notice relating to prescribing, supply, etc. of drugs.	(a) Summary (b) On Indictment		—	—	6 months or £2,000 or both. 2 years or a fine, or both.

eighteen with glues, solvents and allied substances. Those convicted under this legislation may receive a six month prison sentence.

Illegal drug dealing can be hugely profitable. In order to attack such profits the Drug Trafficking Offences Act (1986) was introduced. This gave the British courts power to confiscate from bank accounts and other sources money and goods identified as being the proceeds of illegal drug trafficking. Those failing to comply with confiscation orders are subject to a sliding scale of prison sentences related to the amounts of money in default. A person failing to pay amounts exceeding £1,000,000 may be imprisoned for ten years.

Under the *Misuse of Drugs (Notification of and Supply to Addicts) Regulations* 1973, doctors are required to supply the Chief Medical Officer at the Home Office with details of persons they believe or suspect to be dependent on opiates, cocaine and allied drugs.

Police powers

Under Section 6 of the *Dangerous Drugs (Prevention of Misuse) Act* (1967) the police were empowered to stop and search without warrant any individual who was 'reasonably suspected' of being in unlawful possession of drugs. These powers of search without warrant also apply to vehicles and vessels. The police may seize and retain any evidence of a drug offence. The position in relation to searching buildings is different. The police may, of course, search premises with the permission of the occupants; otherwise a search warrant is required. Police with such a warrant are authorised to enter premises, if necessary by force. It is an offence to obstruct the police in their efforts to seek evidence of a drug offence. 'Obstruction' has been interpreted by the courts to include anything to impede the police, including swallowing the evidence. Under the *Misuse of Drugs Act* (1971) the police were given additional powers of arrest if they had reasonable grounds for expecting that person to abscond, or if they could not dependably establish an individual's real name and address.

An important constraint upon the wide police powers to stop and search was imposed by Home Office Circular Number 133 in 1971. This directive stated that 'modes of dress and hairstyle alone should never, by themselves or together, be regarded as reasonable grounds to stop and search'. Even so, refusal to co-operate with such searches is a crime and there is little doubt that individuals with conspicuous, eccentric or bizarre appearances might be particularly likely to attract the attentions of the police.

Sentencing of drug offenders

The great majority (roughly five out of six) of people convicted of *possessing* controlled drugs are fined or given some form of non-custodial sentence.

More than half of those individuals convicted of 'drug pushing', the production, supply, import and export of controlled drugs, are given custodial sentences. In addition, about an eighth of those convicted of cultivating cannabis plants receive a custodial sentence. Most of these sentences relate to cannabis. It is clear that enormous regional differences exist between the sentencing policies of magistrates, judges or sheriffs. In some areas (such as the Lake District) convictions for possession of cannabis may lead to minimal fines, while elsewhere (such as the Channel Islands) the same convictions may result in a six month prison sentence. Such perplexing variations are not unique to the field of drug control, but they do exemplify the range of differing local attitudes to the seriousness of cannabis smoking and related practices.

Alcohol and tobacco

Western society's two most widely used (and heavily taxed) drugs are subject only to minimal controls in Britain. *Tobacco* may be freely distributed without licence. The only real restriction is that all tobacco products must carry Government health warnings. In addition, tobacco products are labelled to indicate their high, medium or low tar content. Under the *Protection of Children (Tobacco) Act* (1986) it is a criminal offence to sell tobacco to persons under the age of sixteen.

Alcohol use and distribution is subject to much wider controls. Licensing laws regulate when and where alcoholic drinks may be sold and other laws relate to drunkenness and drunken driving.

Licensing laws

The present system of alcohol licensing was introduced during the First World War. These Regulations were intended to restrain alcohol consumption by strategically vital munitions workers and so aid the war effort. Alcoholic drinks can only legally be sold in licensed premises. Different types of licences exist for pubs, restaurants, clubs and other retailers. Special licences may also be obtained for specific occasions such as dinners, dances and conferences.

Before 1976 liquor licensing hours in Scotland were more restricted than they were in England and Wales. Liquor licensing arrangements were reviewed by two committees. One of these related to England and Wales (Erroll 1971) and the second related to Scotland (Clayson 1972). Both of these committees adopted a 'social integrationist' approach and recommended that current licensing hours should be extended in the hope that this would serve to make bar room drinking more relaxed. In the event none of the Erroll Committee's recommendations on longer hours were enacted. Scottish opening hours were, however, extended. The *Licensing (Scotland) Act* (1976) introduced three main innovations. Since December 1976 public bars have been permitted to remain open after 10 pm (their original closing time). Subsequently public houses have also been allowed to open on Sundays. Before this change Sunday opening was only legal for bars in restaurants, hotels and licensed clubs. 'All day licences', regular extensions of permitted bar room hours, were introduced in 1977. A review of these changes has indicated that they have had little impact on alcohol-related illness and death (Duffy and Plant 1986). At the time of writing a debate is continuing about the advisability of introducing flexible opening hours for bars in England and Wales. In England Sunday opening hours (which also cover public holidays, Christmas Day and Good Friday) are from 12 noon–2 pm and from 7 pm–11 pm. In Wales the Sunday hours are the same as they are in England in counties where Sunday drinking is allowed. This is decided by local polls which occur every seven years (the next is due in 1989). As the result of the 1982 poll only two of the 37 Welsh areas do not allow Sunday drinking.

In many areas hours of permitted sale may on occasion be extended if for any special reason a 'late licence' is deemed appropriate – for example, for special social functions. In addition, one can usually buy alcohol in a licensed restaurant provided it accompanies a meal.

Licensed clubs throughout Britain may obtain permission to sell alcohol virtually unhindered during their normal opening hours. In addition, off-licences, wine shops, supermarkets and other establishments may also obtain licences for the sale of alcohol off their premises. Recently there has been a notable increase in the sales of alcoholic beverages through supermarkets and similar outlets.

The quantities of alcoholic drinks sold in pubs are regulated by law and it is an offence to be served in short measure. Spirits are sold in one-sixth gill in England and Wales and one-fifth gill in Scotland. Draught beer and cider are sold in pints or half pints and canned beers, etc. have to be labelled so that their contents are clearly stated. Wines, fortified wines and vermouth do not have to be sold in specific measures and the size of a 'glass' of such beverages varies accordingly.

Young people in licensed premises

A number of rules restrict the access of young people to licensed premises or to alcoholic beverages. Except with the authority of a doctor or in a medical emergency it is an offence to give intoxicating liquor to a child under the age of five, even in the home. It is also an offence to allow a child under the age of fourteen into a bar or licensed premises, including places where alcohol is sold under an occasional licence during permitted hours. Children should not be in bars; even so they *may* be allowed in rooms where alcohol is only either sold *or* consumed, such as off-licence premises or a room in a hotel where people drink alcohol but do not buy it. Young people aged fourteen and over may be allowed in any part of licensed premises, including bars, subject to the licensee's discretion and provided they do not consume alcoholic drinks.

Licensees of pubs may, if they choose, refuse admission to any person provided this does not infringe laws such as those against racial or sexual discrimination.

Laws on drunkenness

It is an offence to be drunk in a public place. In practice people are only arrested if, in addition to being drunk, they are noisy or otherwise behave in an anti-social way. In England and Wales the relevant offences are termed 'drunkenness' and 'drunk with aggravation'. In Scotland such offences are classified as 'drunk and incapable'. The majority of drink-related offences are in connection with the *Road Traffic Act* (1972) which makes it illegal to be unfit to drive a car due to the influence of alcohol, drugs or a combination of both. In addition, this legislation also makes it an offence to be in charge of a bicycle, a horse or a child when under the influence of alcohol or drugs. Most people convicted under this legislation are charged with driving while over the legal blood alcohol or breath alcohol levels.

The police are allowed to stop motorists if they have *reasonable grounds* for suspicion that they are drunk. Suspects will be asked to provide a sample of breath which is analysed by a Lion Auto-Alcometer. The maximum legal limit using this device is 35 micrograms of alcohol in 100 millilitres of breath. Most of those prosecuted record over 40 micrograms. Those whose level is below 50 micrograms have a statutory right to demand either a blood or urine sample if they so choose. These procedures were elaborated in the *Transport Act* (1981). The legal maximum limit for drinking and driving is 80 milligrams of alcohol to 100 millilitres of blood. This is a much *higher* level than that enforced in some countries. In Norway, for example, it is illegal to drive while *any* alcohol is detectable in urine. It is also an offence to be drunk in charge of a stationary vehicle, as long as it is on a public road. People can therefore be convicted of 'sleeping it off' in parked cars if their blood alcohol levels are above the legal limit. It is worth noting that the great majority of people will have their abilities to drive severely reduced well before the fairly liberal legal limit of 80 mgms %. The maximum penalty for drunken driving is a fine of £2000 and/or six months in prison. Conviction now carries automatic disqualification from driving. At present there is no 'breathalyser' in use to detect the influence of drugs apart from alcohol. Even so, the law is often interpreted fairly liberally. For example, in 1979 two individuals were convicted of a breach of the peace in Oban, Argyll. The offenders were alleged to be under the influence of glue.

One alcohol-related problem which has caused widespread public and political concern during recent years is football hooliganism. The *Criminal Justice (Scotland) Act* (1980) restricted the carriage, sale and consumption of alcohol at sporting events, specifically football matches and on transport (e.g. trains and coaches) associated with sporting events. These measures have been widely applauded. In 1985 Liverpool City football supporters attending a match at the Heysel Stadium in Brussels were involved in an allegedly drunken rampage which left 48 people dead. This event, which was a major national and international scandal, led to the speedy introduction of the *Sporting Events (Control of Alcohol etc.) Act* (1985). Following the example of the earlier Scottish legislation this controlled the use and supply of alcohol in sports grounds in England and Wales and on sports-related transport. At the time of writing a number of football clubs appear to be slithering through loopholes in the 1985 Act in order to boost their bar profits. In spite of this legislation, violence by drunken football fans continues to be a serious problem. It must be noted that this is not solely a British phenomenon.

Prescribed drugs

British legislation governing the production and distribution of medicines dates from 1540. In that year an Act was passed that empowered the Royal College of Physicians in London to appoint inspectors to examine 'apothecary wares, drugs and stuffs'.

During the nineteenth century further legislation penalised the adulteration of drugs and the *Therapeutic Substances Act* (1925) was introduced to govern the manufacture of sera, vaccines and hormones.

Before 1964 drugs could be marketed without having to pass any independent standards of safety. The Thalidomide tragedy (which was avoided in America thanks to a commendable refusal to allow the drug to be used) led to the establishment of the Committee on Safety of Drugs (the Dunlop Committee) in 1964. This body was entrusted with the responsibility of vetting drugs and evaluating their safety. In 1965 the Committee of Enquiry into the Relationship of the Pharmaceutical Industry and the National Health Service (the Sainsbury Committee) was set up. It was highly critical of the methods of drug advertising, which, it concluded, were often more concerned with promoting the product than with conveying accurate information. The Sainsbury Committee recommended that an independent and impartial Medicines Commission should be established which would have the widest powers of approving and licensing medicines for sale in the

United Kingdom. The *Medicines Act* (1968) resulted from these recommendations, which replaced the Dunlop Committee with the Committee on Safety of Medicines. In addition, a Medicines Commission was set up to advise the Government. The Act further required pharmaceutical companies to obtain licences for drugs before they could be imported, exported or sold, and further compelled such companies to supply doctors with objective information about their products. The *Medicines Act*, like the *Misuse of Drugs Act* (1971) described above, classified the substances it covered into three groups. First, there are prescription-only medicines. These are substances which are identified as requiring medical supervision because of possible dangers of misuse. Substances likely to cause dependence, such as the opiates, are in this category. Second, some medicines can be sold without prescription, but only by a qualified chemist. Third, there is a general list of medicines which can be sold anywhere. These include laxatives and mild cough mixtures.

The controls permitted by the *Medicines Act* (1968) are currently defined under the *Medicines (Prescription Only) Order* (1977) which came into operation on 1 February 1978. This Order, which applies throughout the United Kingdom, outlines the precise conditions under which a considerable range of medicines may be prescribed or otherwise supplied. The range of preparations available only on prescription was further extended later during the same year under the *Medicines (Prescription Only) Amendment (No. 2) Order* (1978) which came into operation on 11 August 1978. These Orders list not only the numerous medicines now available only on prescription given by a doctor, a dentist, a veterinary surgeon or a veterinary practitioner but also certain exemptions specified for people such as professionals who require special access to drugs (such as agricultural analysts, pharmacists and registered ophthalmic opticians). Legislation controls the maximum strength of dosage and the purpose, pharmaceutical form and route of administration permitted for each controlled medicine. In addition, requirements are specified for prescriptions (including repeat prescriptions, signature and date of signature).

A widely accepted anomaly in the present drug control laws is the virtual lack of control over barbiturates which can produce dependence just as easily as the opiates. While the Campaign on Use and Restriction of Barbiturates (CURB) has successfully led to a great reduction in the prescribing of these drugs, a black market in them still flourishes, apparently partly supplied from over-prescribing. While the *Misuse of Drugs Act* (1971) did not originally prohibit the supply or possession of barbiturates, individuals have been convicted of selling them under Section 58 of the *Medicines Act* (1968). This legislation prohibits any person from selling medicines without a medical practitioner's licence if the commodity in question should only be available on prescription. It is clear that the 1968 Act was not intended to apply to illegal drug trafficking. The use of the *Medicines Act* for such almost certainly helped to extend the *Misuse of Drugs Act* (1971) to cover barbiturates.

As this chapter describes, a very wide range of psychoactive substances are currently subject to some restrictions related to their production or supply. Some substances are not so controlled. Glues and solvents are relatively freely available in spite of some legal controls on their supply because they are in common use for 'legitimate' purposes unrelated to their mood-altering properties. Unprepared psilocybe 'Liberty Cap' mushrooms are not covered by legal restraints, nor are other potentially mood-altering substances such as nutmeg.

Alcohol and tobacco have long been used on a large scale in many countries. In consequence, they are not, whatever the problems of their misuse, subject to anything like the restrictions imposed upon other drugs adopted or even invented more recently. One wonders how either of these two popular recreational substances would fare if subjected to the same stringent criteria of evaluation as newly invented drugs. Would tobacco, or even alcohol, be made freely available for human consumption? Clearly each society has its own system of assessing the advantages and disadvantages of specific forms of drug use. Such assessments have much more to do with tradition and social attitudes than with an 'objective' comparison of the chemical effects of each specific substance.

5 Patterns of Drugtaking

Much more is known about the use of some drugs than others. Substances that are legally produced, distributed and used are relatively well documented. The brewers, distillers, tobacco and pharmaceutical companies are taxed and the scale of their output is recorded. Illegal drug production, distribution and use is, for obvious reasons, harder to gauge. Illicit drug use includes not only substances such as cannabis and heroin but also illegal distilling which, although rare, apparently still sometimes occurs. In addition, the extent of the use of indigenous fungi and other forms of vegetation as psychoactive drugs, or of glues and solvents for similar purposes, is far from clear. Very often it is difficult to obtain a dependable picture of the general extent of the use of a particular drug. It is doubly difficult, as explained in the following chapter, to acquire information about the extent of drug *misuse*, or of drug dependence.

Legal drug production and distribution

A considerable amount of information is available about the amounts of alcohol, tobacco products and prescribed drugs that are produced by their respective industries. This information enables *overall trends* to be measured in relation to the whole population. For example, it is possible to compare annual levels of average alcohol and tobacco consumption by relating the total sales of these commodities to the size of the population. Similarly it is possible to compare either the output of the pharmaceutical industry or the number of psychoactive drug prescriptions during different years. Such information indicates the general levels and trends of drug consumption. It does not, in itself, reveal what percentage of people use drugs, or how levels of drug consumption vary between different sub-groups of the population or within the entire population. If the average level of alcohol consumption per head of the population doubles over a period it does not follow that everyone drinks twice as much. Some people do not drink at all while others become relatively heavy drinkers. In addition it is possible that some groups, such as teenagers or females, may in fact increase their consumption by much more than certain other groups.

A further complication is that overall levels of drug consumption do not necessarily in themselves indicate the extent of drug-related problems. Some people are more vulnerable to the effects of drugs than others by virtue of their weight, sex, general health, mental and social characteristics. Some people may get aggressive after a few drinks, while others do not. These factors are amplified in the next chapter. It does not follow that those purchasing drugs or having drugs prescribed for them necessarily use them. In addition, official records of alcohol and tobacco consumption do not include supplies that countless tourists bring into the country after trips abroad. Conversely, considerable quantities of alcohol and tobacco are consumed not by the resident population but by visitors from overseas who are not taken into account when official levels of average consumption are calculated.

Surveys

Surveys are the main sources of information about the levels of drugtaking behaviour within the population. The drink and tobacco industries routinely carry out their own market research studies to examine who buys their products and in which parts of the country they sell best. In addition, there have been surveys mounted by academic researchers and by Government agencies. The Family Expenditure Survey regularly examines how much families report spending on alcohol and tobacco. There have been several large-scale surveys of drinking and smoking habits. Most surveys have been relatively small-scale affairs limited to specific areas or to highly unrepresentative populations such as school pupils, students or to people in single occupations. Such specific studies are of great value, but they clearly do not form a basis for generalisation to the overall community.

The besetting limitation of surveys of drug use is that people appear to *under-report* their real consumption. Evidence suggests that respondents to surveys often give what they regard as socially respectable answers, sometimes providing the types of reply for which they believe the researchers are hoping. People sometimes over-report their drug use when responding to surveys. There is some evidence that those most likely to over or under-report their drug use are those who are in reality the heaviest users. Apart from intentional deception, people often genuinely forget what their precise drug use has been. Can *you* recall *exactly* what you have had to smoke or drink during the past week? Possibly you could not, especially if the past week involved a riotous party or other similar occasion.

Population surveys are usually dependent for their coverage on the Electoral Register or some other list of possible respondents. Such lists become quickly outdated and generally exclude those with no fixed abode, people who are briefly visiting the study area, those whose jobs involve frequent travelling, students, hospital patients, prisoners and those in other institutions. In addition survey results are commonly limited by a considerable level of non-response. Some people, often 5% at least, *refuse* to provide information about their drinking and smoking habits, let alone their use of illegal drugs. Apart from those who refuse to co-operate other respondents are simply not contacted because they are out when interviewers visit them. It is possible that people excluded from surveys may differ in important ways from those who are contacted and who agree to co-operate. Non-contacts and refusal often comprise well over 10% of those selected for inclusion in surveys. Some of those who, for whatever reasons, are excluded from survey coverage may be especially important in relation to drug use since some sections of the community use both legal and illegal drugs much more than others.

Other sources of information

Some useful insights into how, when and why people use drugs are available from *autobiographical accounts* by drug users. Some of these, notably the writings of Aleister Crowley, Aldous Huxley, Timothy Leary and William Burroughs, are quite well known and have often been quoted as authoritative sources of information. Such accounts are inevitably subjective and may not form a basis for drawing more general conclusions. Even so, one cannot appreciate the many facets of legal and illegal drug use and misuse from shallow statistics. Percentages may indicate levels or trends but do not explain how people feel about drugs or convey much idea of their real significance in society. It is of crucial importance how drug use in its many forms is perceived and why it is indulged in by the drugtakers themselves. Their accounts might be biased, but they cannot justifiably be ignored. Similar insights into how drugs are used in the community are provided by *observation studies* of drugtakers in their natural settings. Such studies certainly have helped to 'pad out' knowledge about drug use and lifestyles associated with it. They too are limited by the observer's biases and inadequacies and such studies are inevitably restricted to quite small, and invariably unrepresentative, groups of people.

Drinking habits

Government departments record annual statistics of total or average alcohol production and sales. In most industrial countries, such figures provide a useful guide to trends in alcohol use. Official figures, as noted above, do not include illicit or unofficial alcohol production which in some countries, such as Norway, is certainly quite extensive. It is generally agreed that very little alcohol is made illegally in Britain, so the official statistics account for the vast bulk of alcohol produced and consumed.

Recent international trends

Alcohol consumption has increased enormously in many countries since the Second World War. This is shown by Table 5.1.

As indicated by Table 5.1, the levels of alcohol consumption in different countries vary enormously. In 1983 the average French person consumed over twice as much alcohol as the average Briton and nearly four times as much as the average Norwegian. Although between 1950 and 1983 alcohol consumption rose in twenty five of the countries cited, it declined in France. In many countries alcohol consumption has either stabilised or has declined during the past few years. This is due to a number of factors, not the least of which has been the recession. Alcohol consumption in the UK reached its post war peak of 7.5 litres of pure alcohol per head of population in 1979 and declined to 6.7 litres in 1982. It rose to 7.0 litres during 1984.

British drinking habits

While alcohol consumption in Britain, like that in many other countries, has risen steadily and by a considerable amount during the past two decades, it remains quite low by international standards. As Table 5.1 illustrates, the highest level of consumption is evident in countries such as France, Spain and Portugal, where wine is the most popular type of alcoholic beverage.

British drinking patterns have undergone some significant changes during recent years. As shown in Table 5.1, between 1950 and 1983 per capita alcohol consumption increased by 92%. The consumption of some types of beverage rose by much more than others. Between 1956 and 1978 per capita beer consumption by those aged fifteen and above in the United Kingdom rose by 47%. The corresponding increases in consumption of spirits and wines were much greater, 153% and 308% respectively. The increase in spirits and wine consumption was especially great during the period 1969–74.

There is no doubt that British drinking habits have become more cosmopolitan, possibly due to the combined effects of advertising and popularity of holidays abroad. This is reflected by a demand for a much greater diversity of drinks, be they imported or home produced. Even so, beer continues to be by far the most popular form of alcohol beverage in the UK, accounting for roughly 60% of all alcohol consumed therein. In the year ending 31st March 1985 the average person in the UK consumed 192.5 pints of beer and 9.4 pints of cider.

Table 5.1 *Per capita alcohol consumption in twenty six countries (1950 and 1983)*

Country*	Per Capita Consumption in Litres of Pure Alcohol		Percentage Change
	1950	1983	1950–1983
Austria	4.8	11.7	+ 143
Australia	6.6 (1981)	5.4	− 22
Belgium	5.4	10.7	+ 98
Bulgaria	4.5 (1960)	14.8	+ 228
Canada	4.4	8.5	+ 93
Czechoslovakia	6.1	11.7	+ 92
Denmark	3.8	10.7	+ 182
Finland	2.2	6.5	+ 195
France	18.7	14.8	− 26
Germany, East	1.5	14.2	+ 846
Germany, West	3.3	12.3	+ 273
Ireland	3.7	6.1	+ 65
Italy	9.5	12.4	+ 30
Japan	3.4 (1960)	5.9	+ 73
Netherlands	2.1	8.7	+ 314
New Zealand	4.4	7.8	+ 77
Norway	2.2	3.8	+ 73
Poland	3.1	6.5	+ 109
Portugal	10.8 (1960)	13.2	+ 22
Spain	8.9 (1960)	12.5	+ 40
Sweden	3.9	5.4	+ 39
Switzerland	8.5 (1960)	10.9	+ 28
USA	5.4	8.2	+ 52
USSR	3.7 (1960)	6.1	+ 65
United Kingdom	3.6	6.9	+ 92
Yugoslavia	4.3 (1955)	8.2	+ 91

* In alphabetical order
Source: Thurman 1986

Several surveys of drinking habits have been carried out in Britain and these have mainly been confined to specific areas such as Camberwell or Clydebank. Several recent studies have had a wider geographical coverage. It is clear that there are some local variations in drinking habits. The Family Expenditure Surveys have shown that Scots spend rather more on alcohol (and tobacco) than either the English or Welsh, but that this difference is not great. A 1976 survey of drinking habits in four Scottish towns indicated that there were quite large variations in the percentage of the adult population who reported drinking or who claimed to be abstainers. In the four towns surveyed (Aberdeen, Ayr, Glasgow and Inverness) the percentage of those interviewed in each town reporting that they were total abstainers ranged from 7% in Inverness to 15% in Glasgow. A more recent survey of drinking habits in the Highlands, Tayside and Kent indicated that while some regional variations were evident, these were relatively minor (Crawford and Plant 1986).

Over 90% of adults in England, Scotland and Wales drink alcohol, even if only occasionally. In contrast, in both Northern Ireland and Eire over a third of adults report being abstainers. A number of surveys have indicated that, contrary to popular belief, alcohol consumption levels in Scotland are not markedly different from those elsewhere in Britain. This is illustrated by Table 5.2.

As Table 5.2 shows, the level of alcohol consumption reported by males in Northern Ireland was lower than that elsewhere in the UK. As the table also illustrates, males typically report drinking two or three times as much alcohol in a week as females. A study of self-reported drinking habits in Trent, East Anglia, Merseyside and the Northern regions of England also indicated that clear regional variations in alcohol consumption existed. Even so these were not nearly as marked as the conventional stereotype of the heavily drinking Northerner suggests (Breeze 1985a).

As already noted, per capita alcohol consumption declined slightly between 1979 and 1984. It is not clear what the general trend of national alcohol consumption has been within different groups of the population. A Scottish survey by the Office of Population Censuses and Surveys (1985) indicated that between 1976 and 1984 alcohol consumption amongst males remained virtually unchanged, while that amongst females rose by over a third. Kendell, De Roumanie and Ritson (1983) noted a small fall in the alcohol

Table 5.2 *Average previous week's consumption* amongst those who consumed alcohol in this period.*

Country	Males Aged 20 or over	Females Aged 20 or over
England and Wales	19.6	7.0
Scotland	19.5	6.2
Northern Ireland	14.5	6.5

* In units of alcohol as defined in Fig. 2.1.
Source: Wilson 1980b

consumption of a study group of men in the Lothian Region between 1978–79 and 1981–82.

It has been widely reported that alcohol consumption by women has risen considerably. This is certainly reflected by the increased consumption of wines, spirits and special lagers, all of which are especially popular among females. Recent market research suggests that over 80% of men prefer beer while two thirds of women prefer other types of alcoholic beverage. There is evidence that the attitudes to drinking of teenage girls are now very close to those of teenage boys. As is described in Chapter 6, trends in alcohol-related problems amongst females have been roughly parallel to those amongst males. There is no doubt that it is far more acceptable now than formerly for females to drink either alone or with others, in public or in private. In addition there are now licensed supermarkets and other retail outlets that permit women to purchase alcoholic drinks without becoming conspicuous.

One reason for the increased level of alcohol consumption in Britain is that in relation to average earnings, alcoholic drinks have become *cheaper*. In 1950 a male manual worker in Britain had to work 23 minutes to earn the price of a pint of beer and 6½ hours to afford a bottle of whisky. By 1976 a pint of beer could be afforded after only 12 minutes and a bottle of whisky after only two hours.

The heaviest drinking section of the population are young working-class men. Dight's Survey of Scottish Drinking Habits revealed that 30% of the alcohol reportedly consumed by the sample of people interviewed had been drunk by only 3%. These were male manual workers in their teens and twenties. Young single people of either sex generally drink more than other older or married people. In addition, manual workers are more likely than non-manual workers to be abstainers. They are also more likely to be heavy drinkers.

A significant feature of British drinking habits is that a very high proportion of alcohol consumption occurs at weekends. A survey of drinking habits in Camberwell carried out in 1965 indicated that drinkers consumed twice as much alcohol on each weekend day (Friday, Saturday and Sunday) as on other days (Edwards *et al.* 1972). A second survey in the same area in 1974 revealed that mid-week consumption had doubled, while that during weekends had changed very little. It is still true that drinking during weekend days is rather greater than during the week, but drinking habits have changed. A more 'Continental pattern' is evident, with a much wider range of beverages being consumed throughout the week and more often at home.

The 1972 Survey of Scottish Drinking Habits confirmed the popularity of weekend drinking:

'The most popular day for drinking is Saturday when nearly three-quarters (of male regular drinkers) had a drink. Over half of the male regular drinkers had a drink on Friday while over 40% had a drink on Sunday. For female regular drinkers the order of preference is the same with 64% having a drink on Saturday, 32% on Friday and 29% on Sunday' (Dight 1976).

Learning to drink

Alcohol is part of the family environment for most people in Britain. Even six-year-olds are often able to identify alcoholic drinks as being different from other beverages. Traditionally boys have been given far more encouragement to drink than girls. This has been changing and the gap between the sexes in this respect appears to have narrowed considerably. Most young children learn about drinking from their parents or from other adults. Usually this helps them to imitate sensible, moderate alcohol use. The influence of home wanes among teenagers who are much more influenced by others of their own age. Drinking is widely accepted as a symbol of sociability and maturity and there is enormous peer pressure among young people to begin drinking. There is no doubt that the vast majority of young people begin to drink alcohol (or to use other drugs) to be sociable and to some extent because of curiosity. Not all parents encourage their children to drink. A minority vigorously disapprove of alcohol use and actively discourage their children from indulging in it. Surveys of school pupils suggest that regardless of parental advice, the overwhelming majority of young people begin to drink before they are legally old enough to purchase drinks in public bars. In addition there is some evidence to suggest that those teenagers most likely to drink heavily include those forced by parental disapproval to use alcohol furtively and outside their own homes.

Tobacco Smoking

Before the mid nineteenth century tobacco was almost exclusively used by males. It was mainly smoked in pipes but was also chewed or taken in the form of snuff. Since the end of the nineteenth century cigarettes have been the popular form in which tobacco is used. Today over 95% of tobacco in Britain is smoked in cigarette form. Smoking among women only became acceptable and widespread after the First World War. Post-war trends in tobacco smoking have been summarised in the Royal College of Physicians (RCP) third report on smoking.

> 'Since 1950, the trend in adult cigarette consumption has been quite different in men and women. Amongst men, a slight upward trend was reversed after 1962, the year in which the first RCP Report was published. The downward trend continued till 1965 since when there has been an upward move, apart from the brief falls after the 1971 RCP Report and tax

increases in 1974, 1975 and 1976. In women a steady upward trend has continued throughout the period, their average consumption rather more than doubling.'

This comment was published in 1977. Between 1972 and 1982 the proportion of smokers in the adult population of Britain *declined*. This was in marked contrast to the general increase in alcohol consumption noted above. As the preceding quotation from the RCP third report suggests, two probable contributing factors were the earlier RCP reports, which publicised the enormous health risks associated with tobacco smoking, and price increases.

Between 1972 and 1982 the percentage of people aged sixteen and above who smoked fell from 46% to 35%. Leck *et al*. (1985: 28) have noted that it has been estimated that by 1984 the proportion of smokers had dwindled to 31%. Between 1972 and 1982 the proportion of male smokers had declined from 52% to 38%. The corresponding fall amongst females was from 42% to 33%.

There is little doubt that public perceptions of smoking have changed during the past decade. Significantly the Chancellor of the Exchequer has recently increased the price of tobacco in the Budget specifically as a *health* measure. Recent surveys show that there is strong public support to ban certain forms of tobacco advertising and to prohibit smoking in public places such as restaurants and cafes. Non-smoking areas have become far more commonplace in cinemas, theatres and on public transport and smoking has been completely banned in London tubes and tube stations. During the 1960s the request, 'Do you mind if I smoke?' was invariably answered with an obliging, 'No, I will find you an ash tray'. Today this is no longer the case and many non-smokers no longer feel obliged to accept the pollution of the air of their homes by guests who do smoke. In California during 1979 a referendum was held on the famous 'Proposition 5'. This measure aimed at prohibiting smoking in a wide range of public places. The proposition was rejected, but its very existence bears evidence of a big shift in public opinion about smoking in some Western countries.

The overall fall in prevalence appears to be mainly due to a consistent decrease throughout the period in the very similar proportions of both sexes who were 'light' smokers (fewer than twenty cigarettes a day). The proportion of men who were 'heavy' smokers (twenty cigarettes or more a day) rose slightly from 24% in 1972 to 26% in 1974, but by 1978 this had fallen back to the same level as in 1972. However, among women, the proportion of heavy smokers continued to increase until 1976 (from 11% in 1972 to 14% in 1976). The drop in the level of tobacco use has been reflected by a slump in the sale of tobacco products in the United Kingdom. Between 1970 and 1984 the number of manufactured cigarettes sold annually fell from 127,900,000,000 to 99,000,000,000.

Table 5.3 *Prevalence of cigarette smoking among males aged sixteen and over in Britain (1972–82)*

	1972	1974	1976	1978	1982
	%	%	%	%	%
Current smokers					
Light (under 20 a day)	28	25	22	22	20
Heavy (20 or more a day)	24	26	24	23	18
Total current smokers	52	51	46	45	38
Ex-regular smokers	23	23	27	27	30
Never or only occasionally smoked	25	25	27	29	32

Source: Office of Population Censuses and Surveys (1979, 1984)

The separate trends among males and females during the period 1972–82 are shown in Tables 5.3 and 5.4.

During the 1970s quite different trends were evident for males and females. Between 1972 and 1978 the average male aged sixteen and over reduced the number of cigarettes smoked per week by 12%. In contrast the corresponding level of average female consumption *increased* by 3%. These differences are shown in Table 5.5.

The reduction in cigarette smoking by both sexes and all age groups between 1972 and 1984 is shown in Table 5.6. This table confirms that the decline in cigarette use during this period was more pronounced among males than among females.

Table 5.4 *Prevalence of cigarette smoking among females aged sixteen and over in Britain (1972–82)*

	1972	1974	1976	1978	1982
	%	%	%	%	%
Current smokers					
Light (under 20 a day)	30	28	24	23	22
Heavy (20 or more a day)	11	13	14	13	11
Total current smokers	41	41	38	37	33
Ex-regular smokers	10	11	12	14	16
Never or only occasionally smoked	49	49	50	49	51

Source: Office of Population Censuses and Surveys (1979, 1984)

Table 5.5 *Cigarette consumption of people aged sixteen and over in Britain (1972–1982)*

	1972	1974	1976	1978	1982
Average number smoked per person per week					
Males	63	64	59	56	
Females	36	38	38	37	
Average number smoked per smoker per week					
Males	120	125	129	127	121
Females	87	94	101	101	98

Source: Office of Population Censuses and Surveys (1979, 1984)

Throughout the 1970s and early 1980s those least likely to smoke were professionals, both males and females. In general higher status workers have both been least likely to smoke at all and have also been most likely to reduce their level of smoking. Semi-skilled and unskilled manual workers have been the most resistant to changing their smoking habits, especially females. For example, between 1972 and 1982 the percentage of smokers among female

Table 5.6 *Prevalence of cigarette smoking in Britain by age and sex (1972 and 1984)*

Age	Males 1972	Males 1984	Females 1972	Females 1984
16–19	43	31	39	30
20–24	55	41	48	40
25–34	56	40	49	37
35–49	55	40	48	38
50–59	54	42	47	40
60 and over	47	33	25	23
Total 16 and over	52	38	41	33

Source: Office of Population Censuses and Surveys (1979, 1984)

professionals declined from 33% to 21%. The corresponding decline among female unskilled manual workers was only from 42% to 41%.

'The 1978 figures on average weekly cigarette consumption per smoker suggest that the trend towards increased consumption per smoker, among both sexes between 1972 and 1976, may have been halted, particularly among male smokers. Between 1976 and 1978 consumption per male smoker declined for all age groups except for those aged 50–59, and in particular there was a marked fall among male smokers aged under 25. Among women smokers, the pattern of change in consumption between 1976 and 1978 was less clear. There was a slight decline among women smokers aged between 35 and 59, and a noticeable fall among those aged 20–24; but in all the remaining age groups consumption per woman smoker continued to increase although less markedly than between 1972 and 1976' (OPCS 1980).

Geographical variations

While cigarette smoking has for some time been in decline in Britain, it appears that there are considerable regional variations in smoking habits. A review by Bostock and Davies (1979) showed that between 1972 and 1976 a higher percentage of the population in Scotland and in Northern and North Western England continued to smoke than in the South East of England. The differences evident during 1976 are summarised in Table 5.7.

The General Household Survey for 1982 confirmed these general differences. The highest proportion of smokers (42%) was found to be in Scotland and the lowest (30%) in East Anglia (Office of Population Censuses and Surveys 1984).

The nature of these apparent regional variations in smoking behaviour has been consistent with evidence reviewed in the following chapter that rates of both alcohol and tobacco-related problems are particularly high in Northern

Table 5.7 *Percentage of current cigarette smokers in Scotland and three English regions (1976)*

	Scotland	SE England	NW England	N England
All males aged 16+	49.8%	43.5%	50.0%	49.8%
All females aged 16+	42.6%	35.0%	41.9%	42.6%

Source: Bostock and Davies 1979

areas of Britain. As Bostock and Davies suggest, a likely influence of these striking regional variations is 'the tremendous social class imbalance between these two areas of Britain', (i.e. South East England and Scotland). Even in Scotland there has been a striking decline in cigarette smoking. The proportion of adult males who smoke declined from 53% to 50% between 1972–6. Conversely the proportion of females who smoke increased very slightly, from 42.1% to 42.6%. In contrast, the proportion of males smoking in England and Wales fell from 51% to 45%, and the proportion of females fell from 41% to 37%. The striking feature of Scottish smoking habits between 1972–6 was the *increase* in smoking by both female teenagers and elderly women. Set against this the proportion of females aged twenty to forty-nine who smoked declined. Even so, between 1974 and 1976 even the proportion of teenage females and older women who smoked began to fall in line with the more general national trend.

Many young people who begin to smoke do so in imitation of their parents. Sometimes smoking is taken up as early as five years of age. A paradoxical fact is that many smokers state that they wish they could give up the habit. A recent survey revealed that this ambivalence is reflected by the fact that most smokers would support further restrictions of smoking in public places. This is also a move that most non-smokers would favour.

Illicit drugtaking

The term 'illicit drugtaking' is used to include both illegal drugtaking and the legal, though socially disapproved, recreational use of substances such as glues and solvents. Information about such drugtaking is more limited than that about drinking or smoking habits. Plenty of research has been carried out in relation to illicit drug use, but this topic inevitably remains rather murky since all forms of illicit behaviour are harder to illuminate than are licit activities. In the following chapter some of the evidence relating to drugtakers identified by 'official agencies' is reviewed. It must be emphasised that most illegal drug use is discreet and does not lead to such identification. Individuals whose drugtaking brings them to the attention of either the police or treatment agencies are no more typical of drugtakers in general than are problem drinkers in clinics representative of all alcohol consumers. For obvious practical reasons certain areas of illegal drugtaking activity remain shrouded in mystery. It simply is not feasible to discover precisely how many cannabis smokers or opiate injectors there are in the community since the overwhelming majority of such people prefer their activities to pass unrecorded and ensure that their behaviour is private. It is doubtful that one could ever obtain a truly representative sample of illegal drugtakers, and no British study has ever claimed to have produced such a thing. Nevertheless, numerous studies of specific sub-groups of drugtakers have been undertaken and these enable some fairly dependable conclusions to be drawn about the general patterns of experimentation with illegal drugs and related substances such as glues, and about the characteristics of those who report using such things.

Users of illicit drugs, like other groups, are susceptible to changing fashions. Patterns of drugtaking consequently vary a great deal over time. It has sometimes been suggested that drugtakers often restrict themselves to a single substance upon which they are very likely to become psychologically, if not physically, dependent. In fact most illicit drug use appears to be casual and largely experimental. There is abundant evidence to support this conclusion. In addition it is clear that many drugtakers have experimented with several types of drug, and that some are willing to smoke, sniff, swallow or even inject virtually anything, legal or illegal, that is available for such use.

Becoming a drugtaker, as noted in Chapter 3, often constitutes a statement of identification with an admired social group. The form that drugtaking assumes similarly reflects the example, habits and values of one's closest associates and friends, or those whom one chooses as exemplars. People generally use whatever drugs are recommended and accepted by their peers. Executives might favour pink gins, while some groups of teenagers appear to prefer smoking a communal joint of cannabis or inhaling the fumes of heroin. There are many types of drugtaker and great diversity in the forms of illicit drug use favoured by such groups.

General characteristics of illicit drugtakers

Age

Surveys and field research show that illicit drugtakers are overwhelmingly young and that most are in their teens, twenties and thirties. Most British drug surveys have been confined to those of at least secondary school age. In spite of this there is evidence that, although illegal drug use is rare amongst younger children it does sometimes occur and is certainly increasing. Even so it is emphasised that regular or dependent drug use amongst people below secondary school age in Britain (with the possible exception of the use of glues and solvents) is uncommon.

Sex

Males are more likely to use illicit drugs than are females. This difference in fact seems to apply to most forms of illegal or disapproved of behaviour. All British surveys have shown that rates of admitted drug experimentation are much higher among males than among females. Presumably females are by upbringing, if not by natural inclination, more law-abiding or conformist to society's expectations. Even so, illicit drugtaking is by no means solely a male pursuit. Many studies suggest that a quarter of cannabis smokers and other illicit drugtakers are females. An observation study of regular drugtakers in

South Hampshire concluded that 47% of those identified as drugtakers were females. Consistent with the general conclusions that most British drugtakers are males, research from America and other Western countries has suggested that roughly 75% of illicit drug users are males.

Ideology

As noted in Chapter 3, there is evidence that there are distinctive ideological differences between drugtakers and non-drugtakers. The former are especially likely to espouse radical political and religious views. Many British and North American studies have shown that drugtakers often state that they are critical of 'traditional' ideologies and values. As drug use has become more widespread the connection between 'ideology' and drugtaking, noted in the 1960s and early 1970s, has probably become weaker.

Becoming a drug user

As emphasised earlier in this book, most people begin using drugs, whether legally or illegally, for social reasons, often to imitate the behaviour of their associates. Most illicit drugtakers report that they initially used drugs either because they were curious about them or because of the encouragement of their friends. Only a minority of illicit drugtakers appear to be drawn to drug use by problems of various sorts. Most youthful drugtaking is convivial, sociable and a corollary of general leisure behaviour.

The first step in becoming a drugtaker involves acceptance of the idea that drug use is harmless and possibly even beneficial. In addition it requires recognition of drugtakers as an attractive or at least acceptable group of people. If a person regards drugtaking as dangerous and those who practise it as pitiful or repugnant it is hardly likely that drug use will be adopted. Before a person engages in 'deviant' activities it is necessary to accept that they are in fact reasonable and justified. Such a frame of mind is necessary before illicit drugtaking. Invariably drug use is preceded by favourable contacts with established drugtakers. Such exposure may lead to a conversion process:

'When I went to college I met people who were using drugs. They seemed OK. They weren't junkies and I saw drugtakers in a new light after that.'

Such statements are commonplace and many people have emphasised that their initial encounters with drugtakers led them to revise their former beliefs about drugtaking and to redefine it as safe and desirable:

'When I was a kid my parents warned me that people who used drugs were either lost or sick. I used to accept the 'establishment view' that drugs were dangerous. When I met people who smoked (cannabis) I learned that this was rubbish. Alcohol and tobacco are drugs. Some of the illegal drugs are probably a lot safer than the so-called "accepted" drugs.'

It is clear that most young illicit drugtakers have been more influenced by the experience and advice of their peers than by the propaganda and admonitions of those attempting to discourage drug use. In addition, the words of popular songs and activities of some popular cult figures such as rock music idols, lend strong support for drugtaking. There is no doubt that among certain groups of young people there are strong pressures to foster drug use:

'A lot of my friends were smoking dope. They often invited me to try it. I felt left out until I did. I wanted to be part of the scene.'

To many people, becoming a drugtaker is an important event and drug use is regarded as indicative of their general approach to life:

'Being a head (drugtaker) is a way of life. It is where you're at . . . Smoking dope is only *part* of the whole scene. It's much more than getting high.'

While there are great differences between drugtakers, largely attributable to educational and social class variations, there appears to be a rather tenuous *esprit de corps*, a vague sense of solidarity among those using illicit drugs. As stated above, most drugtakers are young and at early stages in their careers. Most appear sociable and are in frequent contact with their peers. They are thereby relatively free to establish their own lifestyles and to express views distinctive of their age and social position. Drugtaking is part of the general social interaction of young adults or aspiring adults. Significantly, many drugtakers report that their first drug experiences followed entry into a new circle of friends, leaving school or moving away from their parental home. Such *rites de passage* are important milestones in a person's life.

The extent of illicit drugtaking

The very fragmented evidence available suggests that different types of illicit drugtakers (e.g. students, factory workers, etc.) vary a great deal in relation to their patterns of drug use. Several British studies have collected information about drugtaking from young people in the community. This evidence makes it clear that most drugtaking is discreet and unobtrusive. Only a small minority of illicit drugtakers come to the attentions of 'official agencies' due to the drug use. As is described in Chapter 6, individuals convicted of drug offences or recorded by drug treatment agencies are far from typical of drug users in general. It is clear that illicit drugtaking is vastly more widespread than Home Office figures suggest. While surveys and other studies provide a useful source of information about the nature and extent of drugtaking they by no means provide an adequate picture and have often been confined to highly selective groups, such as students, who were assumed at the outset to be amenable to drug experimentation.

Binnie and Murdock (1969) carried out a survey of higher education students in Leicester and concluded that 9% had used drugs. They described the 'ideal typical user' as:

> 'a middle class male from London or another large town, in his first year at university, atheist or agnostic, with a tendency to hold left-wing political opinions and regarded himself as an average student academically.'

Wiener (1970) surveyed drugtaking among a sample of British secondary school pupils and concluded that 6% had experimented with illicit drugs. In another survey of secondary school pupils, Hindmarch (1972) found that 10% had used drugs. Surveys of British university students have shown that in some institutions at least 10% have used drugs. Evidence suggests that certain types of students such as those doing social science and arts subjects are more likely to report having used illicit drugs than those doing subjects such as business studies or engineering. A survey of medical students at Glasgow University revealed that 14% admitted having used cannabis, LSD and other illicit drugs (McKay, Hawthorne & McCartney 1973). Another Glaswegian study examined the prevalence of admitted drugtaking among sixteen to twenty-four-year-olds in the following groups: school pupils, college and university students, patients attending special (VD) clinics and casualty patients. Information was collected from 2809 individuals, of whom 31% reported having used illicit drugs (Fish *et al*. 1974). An earlier survey of 305 people aged seventeen to twenty-four living in Cheltenham had revealed that 20% reported having at some time used either cannabis, LSD or amphetamines (Plant 1972).

Kosviner and Hawks (1977) carried out a survey of drug use in two British university colleges. They found that 37% of those in one college and 38% of those in the second reported having used illicit drugs.

The British Crime Survey was undertaken during 1981. This showed that 16% of those aged 20 to 24 in England and Wales and 19% of those of the same age in Scotland had at some time reportedly used cannabis (Chambers and Tombs 1984, Mott 1985).

In 1982 the Daily Mail published the results of a sample survey of self-reported drug use amongst people aged 15 to 21. The results of this survey are shown in Table 5.8.

This study showed that in most areas of Britain 1% of those interviewed reported having used heroin or cocaine and between 13% and 28% reported having used cannabis. It also indicated that the level of youthful drug use in Scotland was particularly high. This conclusion related to very small numbers and may have reflected considerable (and misleading) sample bias.

Between 1979 and 1983 a follow-up study was conducted of the drinking, smoking and illegal drug use of 1,036 young adults in the Lothian Region in South East Scotland. These individuals were aged 15 and 16 when the study started and were aged 19 and 20 during 1983. At the ages of 15 and 16, 15.2%

Table 5.8 *Regional variations in self-reported illicit drug use amongst the 15–21 age group in Britain*

Drugs ever used	Area				
	Scotland	North of England	Midlands, East Anglia, Wales	South of England excluding London	London
	(n = 57*) %	(n = 447*) %	(n = 338*) %	(n = 330*) %	(n = 153*) %
Cannabis	21	15	16	13	28
Amphetamines	8	4	6	3	10
Glues	2	5	1	2	4
Barbiturates	16	2	4	2	3
LSD	8	3	4	2	3
Heroin	7	**	1	1	1
Cocaine	9	1	1	1	3

* weighted total
** less than 0.5%
Source: NOP Market Research Ltd., 1982.

of males and 10.7% of females had reportedly used some form of illicit drug. During 1983, when 92.4% of the study group were re-interviewed, these proportions had risen to 37.0% and 23.2% respectively. This is illustrated by Table 5.9.

The Lothian follow-up study showed that young people who, at the ages of 15 and 16, were heavy drinkers were especially likely to have used illegal drugs by the ages of 19 and 20. Another finding of this study was that levels of illicit drug use were particularly high amongst young unemployed people.

During the 1960s it was evident that illegal drug use was especially prevalent in some areas such as Crawley (de Alarcon and Rathod 1968). Similar local variations are evident today. For example a study of drug problems in Glasgow noted that drug use was particularly commonplace in some of the City's more deprived areas (Haw 1985). A study of the Wirral in Cheshire also indicated a link between problem drug use and social deprivation and suggested that even within this relatively small area, there were over 1,600 problem drug users most of whom used opiates (Parker, Bakx and

Table 5.9 *Changes in self-reported drug use amongst a study group of young people in the Lothian region (1979/80 to 1983)*

Drug	Males (n = 436) 1979/80 n	%	1983 n	%	Females (n = 514) 1979/80 n	%	1983 n	%
Cannabis	32	7.3	152	34.9	35	6.8	114	22.2
LSD	4	0.9	25	5.7	6	1.2	13	2.5
Barbiturates	5	1.1	4	0.9	7	1.4	7	1.4
Mogadon	6	1.4	6	1.4	3	0.6	8	1.6
Librium	1	0.2	3	0.7	2	0.4	3	0.6
Valium	16	3.7	17	3.9	19	3.7	11	2.1
Glues/solvents	20	4.6	10	2.3	20	3.9	8	1.6
Amphetamines	5	1.1	36	8.3	15	2.9	27	5.2
Opium	2	0.5	4	0.9	3	0.6	1	0.2
Morphine	0	—	1	0.2	1	0.2	0	—
Heroin	2	0.5	3	0.7	2	0.4	3	0.6
Methadone	no data		2	0.5	no data		1	0.2
Cocaine	7	1.6	10	2.3	2	0.4	10	1.9
Sleeping tablets/ tranquillisers	20	4.6	9	2.1	27	5.2	8	1.6
PCP (angel dust)	no data		1	0.2	no data		0	—
Hallucinogenic fungi	no data		21	4.8	no data		9	1.8

Source: Plant, Peck and Samuel 1985

Newcombe 1986). Bucknall and Robertson (1986) have reported that a single health centre in the Muirhouse area of Edinburgh has over 160 opiate users on its books. A survey of 2,417 secondary school and college students in England and Wales indicated that 17% had used cannabis, 6% had used solvents and 2% had used heroin (Williams 1986).

The Drug Indicators Project has gathered evidence suggesting that between 20,000 and 30,000 people in the London area were regularly using opiates during 1984 (Hartnoll 1985).

Individual surveys are certainly flawed by bias and provide an imperfect and very narrow picture of the nature and extent of illegal drug use. Taken together the available evidence suggests that drug use has been spreading fairly rapidly during recent years and is currently at an unprecedented level. Those who use drugs include young people in virtually all social positions. Even so, a growing body of evidence suggests that the unemployed and those living in the most deprived areas are especially likely either to use drugs or to develop drug problems (Peck and Plant 1986).

Patterns of illicit drugtaking

Survey data confirm that relatively large numbers of young people have used illicit drugs, but that in most cases such use is very limited. Far fewer people are regular users. Several studies have collected information from such regular users. These suggest first that cannabis is overwhelmingly the most commonly used illicit drug and secondly that many of those who do smoke it regularly have also used other illicit substances. An illustration of such *polydrug use* is provided by three studies, all of which collected information from groups of people professing to be regular cannabis smokers. These groups were interviewed in South Hampshire and Cheltenham in Britain and New York in the USA. The majority of these cannabis smokers stated that they had also used other illicit substances. The range of drugs ever used by the drugtakers in the two British studies is shown in Table 5.10.

Strikingly similar results were produced by the New York study (Goode 1970). This showed that among a group of 204 regular cannabis smokers 49% had used LSD, 43% amphetamines, 13% heroin, 20% opium and 19% cocaine. In fact the patterns of drug use reported by the New York and Cheltenham studies (both of which were confined to regular cannabis smokers) were almost identical. Broadly similar patterns of experimentation are indicated by the more recent studies shown in Tables 5.8 and 5.9.

Cannabis has, for the past two decades, been the mainstay of the drug

Table 5.10 *Drugs ever used by regular illicit drugtakers in two British studies*

Drugs ever used	Cheltenham %	South Hampshire %
Amphetamines	54	70
Hypnotics	46	64
Cannabis	100	98
Raw opiates	16	44
Manufactured opiates	15	48
Hallucinogens	77	76
Cocaine	15	30
Miscellaneous non-medical substances	11	34
Miscellaneous medical substances without prescription	no information	45
Prescribed medicines	no information	33
Total	n = 200	n = 122

Source: Plant and Reeves 1973

scene. As described in the following chapter, this pre-eminence is reflected by the fact that far more people are convicted of possessing cannabis than of any other proscribed drug.

Surveys and field research suggest that within many drugtaking circles considerable prestige is accorded to those who have experimented with a wide range of different substances. In consequence, some 'dedicated' drugtakers report having tried an amazing range of obscure herbs, plants and concoctions as well as virtually every proprietary brand of medicine in search of a new 'buzz' or effect.

While wide-ranging experimentation may often be approved of, it is clear that many illicit drugtakers shy away from the use of opiates or injected drugs. Studies of middle class or better educated groups of drugtakers indicate that drug injection is very rare and that such practices are widely regarded as dangerous and are avoided as such. There appears to be very little support for drug injection among university students. In spite of this it is apparent that heroin and cocaine have sometimes been used in some student circles. Even so, lower-status drugtakers, such as manual workers, often report having used opiates or injected drugs. To a large extent the adoption of such 'extreme' patterns of illicit drugtaking is related to depth of involvement with the drugtaking way of life as opposed to commitment to education and careers. Injection and opiate use seem to be most popular among those with least commitment to the workaday world, low status, unemployed or manual workers. It is not uncommon to find such young people who have taken heroin in a fairly casual fashion, as illustrated by this comment from a West Country building labourer:

> 'Yes, I fixed (injected) a few years back. When I lived in Southampton it was easy to get smack (heroin). Quite a few of us used to fix at weekends. I only did it twice. It's easy to get too much into fixing. I won't do it again. Most of us were disappointed, like.'

Some people do become physically dependent upon illicit drugs. These are described in Chapter 6. The great majority of drugtakers do not become dependent, either because they are not particularly regular users or because they use a wide variety of substances, depending upon which are available and which are regarded as acceptable by their friends. In view of the willingness of many drugtakers to experiment with a profusion of substances the distinction between 'hard' and 'soft' drug use is not really a very helpful one. There are people who, though deeply involved with drugtaking, do not use opiates and others who have used them, but only very casually and without much commitment. The depth and extent of a person's involvement with drugs are at least as significant as the types of drug used.

Most drugtakers restrict their use of drugs so that it does not interfere with their major preoccupations, their education and careers. Most regard drugtaking as one facet of their leisure and not as a central issue.

The association of illicit drugs with alcohol and tobacco

Surveys show that the young people most likely to use illegal drugs are often regular or heavy users of alcohol and tobacco. Very often the heaviest drugtakers are also the heaviest drinkers and smokers. As noted above, the heaviest drinkers in the population are mainly young working-class males. These also appear to be the heaviest smokers and the heaviest and most catholic users of illicit substances. The 'newer' drugs, such as cannabis, are often used in conjunction with alcohol. Indeed, cannabis is invariably smoked in a mixture with tobacco. Young people who smoke and drink appear much more likely than those who do not to try cannabis and other illicit substances. As the American sociologist, Erich Goode commented:

> '. . . people who use illegal drugs, marijuana (cannabis) especially, are fundamentally the same people who use alcohol and cigarettes – they are a little further along the same continuum. People who abstain from liquor and cigarettes are far less likely to use marijuana than people who smoke and/or drink' (Goode 1972).

It seems that alcohol, tobacco and the illicit drugs are not necessarily mutually exclusive. Their contexts of use are similar, as are the reasons why most users take them. The illicit drugs have been blended into youthful leisure along with alcohol and tobacco, even though a big gulf exists between the popularity of the legal and the illicit drugs.

Prescribed drugs

A 1979 British survey revealed that 18% of males and 34% of females report that at some time they have taken sleeping tablets or tranquillisers on prescription (MORI 1979). The scale of such prescribed drug use is enormous, costly and is increasing:

> 'The true increase in psychoactive drug prescription per unit of a standard population over the past twelve years is about 34%, equivalent to a compound annual growth rate of about 2%. At present about 8% of adults in the United Kingdom are on treatment with psychoactive drugs.
>
> But this level of psychoactive drug usage is not confined solely to the United Kingdom. Between one-tenth and one-sixth of the adult population of the United States and . . . Belgium, Denmark, France, (West) Germany, Italy, Netherlands, Spain, Sweden, and the United Kingdom . . . were using sedatives and anti-anxiety drugs in 1971. The difference between the various countries could not be ascribed to factors of religion, social attitudes or to subsidised health care. The main factor in this level of use appears to be loneliness.' (Marks 1978).

The pattern of psychoactive drug prescribing has altered considerably during the past two decades. While there has been a steady rise in the general level of prescribing, the type of drugs most widely used have changed a great deal. During the early 1960s amphetamines (pep pills) were dispensed in large quantities. They represented 2.5% of National Health Service prescriptions in 1961. Concern over their misuse, as noted in Chapter 2, led to a voluntary curtailment of amphetamine prescribing. Barbiturates have had a similar history. They were very widely used until safer alternatives such as Mogadon, Ativan, Librium and Valium were available. Recognition of the dangers of barbiturates, combined with the introduction of preferable substitutes and a vigorous campaign to limit barbiturate prescribing have led to a reduction in barbiturate use. Between 1972 and 1984 the annual number of barbiturate prescriptions in Britain fell from 11,688,000 to 1,914,000. This is shown by Table 5.11. An indication of the levels of benzodiazepine prescribing is provided by Table 5.12.

Table 5.11 *Barbiturate prescriptions in Britain (1972–1984)*

Year	Number of prescriptions (*thousands*)
1972	11,688
1973	10,729
1974	9,616
1975	8,156
1976	6,859
1977	5,997
1978	5,160
1979	4,456
1980	3,595
1981	2,980
1982	2,465
1983	2,303
1984	1,914

These data are estimates based on a sample of prescriptions of 1 in 200 in England and Wales, and 1 in 100 in Scotland, which were dispensed by retail pharmacists and appliance contractors.

Source: Department of Health and Social Security (Personal Communication) (1986)

Table 5.12 *Benzodiazepine prescriptions in Britain (1980 and 1984)*

Drug	Number of prescriptions 1980	1984
Nitrazepam (Mogadon)	9,014	6,403
Diazepam (Valium)	8,819	5,407
Tamazepam (Normison)	1,329	4,222
Lorazepam (Ativan)	2,390	3,240
Flurazepam (Dalmane)	2,300	1,970
Chlordiazepoxide (Librium)	2,156	1,347
Triazolam	544	1,274
Potassium Clorazepate	1,181	1,255
Oxazepam	688	645
Lormetazepam	—	521
Clobazem	326	487
Alprazolam	—	339
Flunitrazepam	—	241
Bromazepam	—	188
Ketazolam	49	158
Medazepam	230	126
Clonazepam	47	90
Loprazolam	—	66
Prazepam	—	65
Total	29,073	28,044

These data are estimates based on a sample of 1 in 200 prescriptions in England and Wales, and 1 in 100 in Scotland which were dispensed by retail chemists and appliance contractors. Brackets give example of brand names. Some benzodiazepines are produced under several brand names.

Source: Department of Health and Social Security (Personal Communication) (1986)

A disproportionate number of those receiving sleeping tablets and tranquillisers are over forty-five years of age. A recent study suggested that 34% of those in this age group have at some time received such drugs on prescription. Even so, a high proportion of younger people also report that they have taken prescribed sleeping tablets or tranquillisers, 28–9% of those aged twenty-five to forty-four and even 13% of those aged fifteen to twenty-four (MORI 1979). Evidence from several Western countries indicates that prescribed tranquillisers are far more likely to be taken by women than by men. This is in marked contrast to male predominance among both drinkers and illicit drugtakers.

Psychoactive drugs are prescribed on a huge scale. There is no doubt that sometimes such prescribing is excessive. In addition, drugs used for overdoses or taken for kicks in the drug scene reflect whatever substances happen to be available currently – amphetamines (1960s), barbiturates (1970s) and benzodiazepines (1980s). The nature and extent of this misuse is discussed in the following chapter. In spite of the abuses that certainly occur, psychoactive drugs appear to be generally dispensed carefully, thoughtfully and with justification. They are of great therapeutic value and the recent trend of replacing barbiturates by much safer alternatives is a welcome development.

6 Drug Problems

The preceding chapter outlined recent evidence relating to the *use* of drugs. While most drug use appears to be moderate and sensible it is abundantly clear that all too often drugs are used excessively or harmfully. In addition it is apparent that the *misuse* of some drugs has been increasing alarmingly during the last few years. In this chapter the extent and distribution of problems related to illegal drugs, alcohol, tobacco and prescribed drugs are reviewed.

As mentioned earlier in this book, one does not need to be physically dependent upon or 'addicted to' a drug to use it unwisely or to suffer harm from its use or to inflict such harm upon others. A considerable proportion of all drug-related damage is attributable to 'being under the effects' of drugs. Bad LSD trips, overdoses and intoxication are obvious examples of the type of harm that can be caused by a single instance of unwise or excessive drug use. Often such acts are just as tragic in their effects as the development over several years of physical dependence. Most drug use, as noted in Chapter 5, is discreet and does not come to the attention of official agencies such as the police or medical services. In addition there is abundant evidence that many people who do use drugs excessively, or who damage themselves because of their drug use, also remain unrecorded. In consequence it is not known how many drug dependants, problem drinkers, etc. there are in the community. The social cost of drug misuse due to accidents, physical disabilities, crimes, violence, industrial absenteeism or inefficiency can only be guessed at. As explained in Chapter 5, surveys of drug *use* appear to produce biased and dubious results. It is even more likely that surveys and other information about drug *misuse* are of limited value in assessing the scale and nature of drug problems.

Many people whose drugtaking causes problems do not seek help from official agencies. In addition there are many views about precisely what constitutes a 'problem' or how one defines a drug misuser or a problem drinker.

In spite of the many scientific difficulties of measuring the extent of drug problems, estimates are all too often publicised. Such estimates are often produced to emphasise that various types of drug misuse are serious social problems deserving greater public or political concern. Sometimes agencies working in the field use such estimates to justify their appeals for financial backing. This reflects the fact that many bodies providing help for drug-related problems are non-statutory and have no guaranteed regular incomes.

The Royal College of Psychiatrists has suggested (1986) that at least 300,000 people in Britain suffer such severe alcohol problems that they justify the label of alcohol dependence. It has been conservatively estimated that alcohol problems in industry annually cost £1,396,000,000 in England and Wales (McDonnell and Maynard 1985). Similarly the Legalise Cannabis Campaign has suggested that as many as 5,000,000 people in Britain have at some time smoked cannabis. In addition it has been speculated that there may be over 80,000 heroin users in Britain. Each of these assessments is plausible. All are at least partly speculative and based upon very limited evidence.

Surveys

As explained in the previous chapter, surveys are an important source of information about the drugtaking habits of the general population. Most surveys have been confined to highly selective samples or to the clients or patients of drug treatment agencies of various types. Very few large scale surveys have been carried out in Britain of alcohol use, let alone that of illegal drugs. Most surveys have been confined to specific areas or to sub-groups of the population which are not representative, even if they are sometimes of particular interest.

Clinical studies

A tremendous amount of information is available from various agencies providing help for people with drug problems. There are literally libraries full of such clinical studies and these provide a very high proportion of the available information about those who become dependent on drugs or who, for other reasons, require help in relation to their drugtaking. Some agencies provide specialist help for those with specific problems, for problem drinkers, opiate dependants, tobacco dependants or for those who have overdosed with drugs. Most statutory agencies routinely record quite a lot of biographical and other information about their clients so that it is possible to describe these in considerable detail. Many non-statutory bodies have extremely limited funds and few, if any, resources to permit research. Others, such as Alcoholics Anonymous, as their name indicates, really are anonymous and often unable or unwilling to keep records of their members' characteristics or subsequent progress.

Clinical studies are invaluable but only relate to known or identified drugtakers. Many, and probably most, of those who use drugs excessively or harmfully do not seek professional help. In consequence most go unrecorded. Population surveys regularly indicate that there are many times more people in the community who do, or who have, experienced drug problems than are known to official agencies. Most problem drinkers, opiate users and others who might possibly interest such agencies do not come forward for help. In consequence it cannot be assumed that clinic populations of drug misusers typify all those in the population who experience drug problems. Certainly they do not. Some people, for example females, may be especially likely to conceal their drug problems because of fear of social stigma. It is also clear that many people who do at some time suffer harmful consequences from drug use do not regard such experiences as particularly devastating or a cause for concern or treatment. Some people appear to be quite happy using drugs 'excessively'.

Drug offences

As described in Chapter 4, the use of many psychoactive drugs is either proscribed or is subject to some legal constraints. A considerable amount of information is available about those convicted of drug offences. These largely relate to substances, such as cannabis, covered by the *Misuse of Drugs Act* (1971) or to public drunkenness and drunken driving. Such data provide profiles of 'who gets into trouble' but do not necessarily tell very much about more general patterns of drug misuse. Only some drunken drivers and people possessing illegal drugs get caught. It is probable that crime statistics only represent a very small part of the picture, just as clinical information does. Official agencies only record information about detected or known drug casualties. While these may well be among those most deeply involved with or harmed by drug use, it does not follow that they are typical or a majority of those in this category. All types of crime data are limited by the so-called 'grey figure' or unrecorded crime, the extent of which is uncertain but probably very large indeed.

Mortality statistics

Sometimes drugtaking has fatal consequences. These may be conspicuous and be recorded as such. Often the link between a death and drug misuse is less apparent and may escape undetected. Liver cirrhosis deaths appear to be *mainly* attributable to excessive drinking, but some are not. A road traffic accident may be due to the use of alcohol or other drugs or to poorly maintained brakes or an icy surface. Many drug-related accidents and deaths, due to the long term effects of drugs on various organs such as the heart or the lungs, fail to be recorded as such. It is known that excessive drinkers run an increased risk of heart disease or that smokers are vastly more at risk of dying from lung cancer than are non-smokers. Most deaths from such causes are not differentiated to reveal the involvement or role of drug use.

Information about the extent of drug problems is limited by the fact that most drug problems are private affairs. Most users of illegal drugs, and most of those dependent upon alcohol, tobacco or prescribed drugs are not identified or recorded as such. In fact very many people in these categories are certainly unaware that their drug use or drug dependence constitutes a problem. Many drug dependent people probably do not realise that they are even dependent or would fervently deny that they were.

Alcohol problems

As noted in Chapter 2, most people appear to drink alcohol sensibly, appropriately and in moderation. Excessive or unwise drinking can lead to a variety of problems or disabilities. These harmful consequences include physical dependence, physical damage and a wide range of social problems. One does not need to be physically dependent upon alcohol to suffer harmful effects from drinking and much of the harm caused by alcohol misuse is attributable to drunkenness and not to dependence upon alcohol. Drinkers may be at any point along a continuum ranging from sensible, harmless drinking at one end to excessive and destructive drinking at the other. While the effects of alcohol depend upon many individual factors such as sex, weight and height, in general the risk of suffering some kind of harmful consequence increases the more a person drinks.

In the preceding chapter it was emphasised that surveys of the *use* of illegal drugs, alcohol and tobacco appear to produce biased and dubious results. It has also been emphasised that most drug use, whether legal or illegal, certainly passes unrecorded by official agencies such as the police, medical services or other bodies providing help for people with drug-related problems. Those recorded by such agencies as casualties are by no means all of those who do develop drug problems and this is likely to apply to the casualties of alcohol use in much the same way as it does to the casualties of illegal drug use. Information about alcohol is available from several sources which together support the conclusion that alcohol problems are in fact extremely commonplace and that they are becoming increasingly so.

Just as surveys provide a considerable amount of information about the drinking habits of the population, they also help to indicate, if only approximately, the nature and extent of alcohol problems among different social groups. As noted in the previous chapter, survey data appear to be highly suspect and are likely to be distorted by considerable under-reporting. Most surveys have been confined to patients or clients attending agencies providing help for alcohol problems. Others have been restricted to atypical sub-groups such as students or members of a specific occupational group. Many studies of alcohol problems have either been confined to males or, until recently, failed to distinguish between the sexes. Only a few surveys of the general population have been carried out and, as noted in the previous chapter, even these have been mainly confined to specific areas.

Alcohol consumption

Figures are available for many countries, as noted in Chapter 5. Alcohol consumption levels are clearly linked to rates of alcohol problems. Even so, such figures do not, in themselves, provide a basis for assessing the extent of alcohol problems in the community or what proportion of people drink excessively.

Clinical records

These are maintained by some agencies providing help for problem drinkers, but not by others. Alcoholics Anonymous and some of the local councils on alcoholism do not keep detailed records. Most problem drinkers certainly remain unknown to such agencies. In addition there is evidence that family doctors identify only a minority of the problem drinkers with whom they have contact. A further complication is that some individuals seeking help or advice for alcohol problems contact several agencies. The numbers of people recorded by treatment agencies depend partly upon the type of help available in a specific area. In general, larger urban areas are the best endowed with such agencies, while in rural districts there may be little specialised help unless a local Alcoholics Anonymous group exists. Many problem drinkers do not live near an agency that would record them even if they contacted it.

Crime statistics

These provide valuable information about drunkenness offences, including drunken driving. As noted above, such figures reflect local police policies and detection methods. As explained in Chapter 4 the definitions of drunkenness offences are different in Scotland from those in England and Wales. Crime figures are also clearly influenced by other factors, such as the numbers of police available to enforce the law and the number of people driving cars, drunk or sober.

Liver cirrhosis deaths

These are widely acknowledged as a useful indicator of the extent of excessive drinking. Approximately three quarters of those dying from this cause in Britain do so as a result of heavy drinking. Even so, only about 12% of known alcohol dependants die from liver cirrhosis. This condition appears to be more likely to develop if an individual drinks daily than only during periodic heavy binges. In consequence some groups of people and countries have rates which, in relation to their general levels of alcohol consumption, are disproportionately high. Liver cirrhosis deaths are a useful indicator of alcohol problems. They do not indicate, however, how many live excessive drinkers there are or how many people indulge in heavy drinking for relatively brief periods that do not cause cirrhosis.

Some recent trends

Both alcohol consumption and rates of alcohol-related problems in the United Kingdom rose during the 1970s. Alcohol consumption has declined slightly since 1979 and in association there has been a decrease in levels of some alcohol-related problems. Some of these trends are indicated by Table 6.1.

The pattern of alcohol-related problems is associated with the rise and fall of alcohol consumption in the general population. In consequence several authorities have concluded that the most obvious way to control the level of alcohol-related problems is to control the general level of alcohol consumption by manipulating the price of alcoholic drinks (Kendell 1979, Central Policy Review Staff 1979, Royal College of Psychiatrists 1986).

Alcohol-related problems are far more extensive than indicated by the evidence cited in Table 6.1. Alcohol misuse is associated with a wide range of accidents, health, social and public order problems. For example the Royal Lifesaving Society has long reported that alcohol is the commonest single factor in drownings, currently featuring in a quarter of such deaths. Many agencies provide help for problem drinkers. These include Alcoholics Anonymous, councils on alcohol problems, Drinkwatchers, community alcohol teams, alcohol problems clinics and a host of non specialist health and social service agencies. The figures in Table 6.1 give no indication of the number of problem drinkers and their relatives who receive help from such agencies, or informally through family and friends.

General characteristics of problem drinkers

The popularly accepted stereotype of the 'alcoholic' is that of a social derelict. In fact, the great majority of people who seek help from agencies for their drinking problems are married, working and have homes. Some problem drinkers are homeless and on 'Skid Row', but these constitute only

Year	UK per capita alcohol consumption in litres of pure alcohol	UK rate of liver cirrhosis mortality*	UK drunkenness convictions*	British drunken driving convictions**	First admissions to British psychiatric hospitals for 'alcoholism', alcoholic psychosis and alcohol dependence*
1970	5.2	3.0	1.7	6.4	6.5
1971	5.5	3.3	1.8	8.9	7.4
1972	5.8	3.5	1.8	10.5	8.1
1973	6.4	3.8	2.0	12.2	9.7
1974	6.7	3.8	2.1	12.6	11.1
1975	6.7	3.9	2.1	12.8	10.7
1976	7.0	4.1	2.2	10.9	10.8
1977	6.8	3.9	2.2	9.9	11.4
1978	7.3	4.2	2.2	11.1	11.1
1979	7.5	4.7	2.4	12.6	11.3
1980	7.2	4.8	2.4	14.4	12.3
1981	6.9	4.8	2.1	13.1	11.6
1982	6.7	4.7	2.1	13.5	10.5
1983	6.9	4.8[a]	2.1[b]	17.6	10.6
1984	7.0	4.9[a]	1.7[b]	18.2	11.3

* Rate per 100,000 total population
** Rate per 10,000 total population
[a] Figure related only to Britain
[b] Figures for England and Wales include cautions

Sources: Thurman 1986, Annual Abstract of Statistics 1979, 1981, 1984, 1985, Home Office Annual Reports, Scottish Home and Health Department annual crime statistics, Brewers Society 1986, Abstract of Statistics 1979, 1981, Health and Personal Social Statistics for England, Health and Personal Social Statistics for Wales, Scottish Health Statistics 1980–1986

a very small percentage, possibly about 5% of those known to be alcohol dependent.

The average age of those seeking help to deal with their drinking problems is the early to mid-forties. However, problem drinking among younger people and, as noted below, among females has become much more commonplace. There are now special facilities in some areas to encourage the young or females to enlist help to overcome their drinking problems. Most of the alcohol problems young people encounter are attributable to intoxication rather than to chronic dependence upon alcohol.

The majority of those who fall foul of the law due to public drunkenness are young male manual workers. As the preceding chapter explained, this group appears to be the heaviest drinking section of the community. Young people are also especially likely to be convicted of drunken driving. This is doubtless partly attributable to their lack of motoring experience, but is clearly also related to their relatively high alcohol consumption. During the past twenty years there was a disproportionate increase in the numbers of young people, especially teenagers, convicted of drunkenness offences. The youthfulness of many of those convicted of such offences contrasts sharply with the greater age of most of those who seek help from agencies for their alcohol problems.

Regional variations

It has long been established that officially recorded rates of alcohol-related problems are higher in the North than in the South of Britain. Several reviews have concluded that the North of England and the North and West of Scotland have markedly higher levels of alcohol-related deaths, illnesses and public order offences than do more southerly regions. Recent evidence suggests that, to a large extent, these differences are due to regional variations in the provision of services for problem drinkers or in methods of recording alcohol-related problems.

As noted in Chapter 5 two studies have examined drinking habits and alcohol-related problems in different areas. One of these related to South East Kent, Tayside and the Highland region (Crawford *et al.* 1984, Latcham *et al.* 1984). The second related to the Merseyside, Northern Trent and East Anglian health regions (Breeze 1985a). Both studies showed that local variations in alcohol consumption did exist. The first study indicated that local variations in drinking habits did not reflect local variations in rates of alcohol-related problems. Moreover it was concluded that the local rates of in-patient admissions for alcohol dependence to psychiatric hospitals did not differ markedly. Official information suggested that the rate of such admissions in the Highland region exceeded that in Kent by over twelve times. Latcham *et al.* (1984) concluded that this apparently huge disparity was in fact quite misleading since far more people diagnosed as alcohol dependent in Kent were treated as out-patients or in non-psychiatric beds. In reality, it was concluded, the alcohol dependence rate in the Highlands exceeded that in Kent by *only* about 50%. Breeze (1985) found that although general alcohol consumption levels in the 'high risk' Merseyside and North of England areas exceeded that in the 'low risk' Trent and East Anglia regions, these differences were not great.

During recent years rates of convictions for public drunkenness and drunken driving in Scotland have been declining in comparison with those in England and Wales. Drunken driving offences appear to have been relatively stable in Scotland, but have been rising south of the border. Public drunkenness offences throughout Britain have been declining, but have recently been at rather higher levels in England and Wales than they have in Scotland. It is probable that this change does not reflect a real Scottish improvement. The *Criminal Justice (Scotland) Act* 1980 led to an extension of the decriminalisation of public drunkenness in Scotland. In consequence some of those who once would have been convicted of alcohol-related public order offences have been referred to detoxification facilities such as the excellent Albyn House in Aberdeen.

It has long been believed that Scotland had higher rates of alcohol-related liver cirrhosis mortality than England and Wales. An examination of this perplexing disparity by Kemp (1986) led to the conclusion that this difference too is largely attributable to variations in the methods of recording such deaths rather than to major differences in the real levels of cirrhosis. Accordingly conventional assumptions about the massive regional variations of alcohol-related problems have been greatly undermined. In spite of this it is emphasised that some regional variations do exist, both in relation to drinking habits and the consequences of alcohol consumption. It is possible that the Scots once drank markedly more than the English, but since surveys of drinking habits are relatively new exercises, this will probably remain a mystery.

Occupational variations

There is abundant evidence that some occupations have particularly high rates of alcohol problems. This conclusion is supported by information from three sources. First, several studies have noted that people referred to agencies providing help for alcohol problems are especially likely to belong to certain occupational groups. Secondly, some studies of specific jobs have noted their high risks of heavy or harmful drinking. Thirdly, certain jobs have extremely high rates of death due to liver cirrhosis. Those jobs with the highest rates are shown in Table 6.2.

Table 6.2 shows sixteen occupational groups in Britain which had the highest rates of death due to liver cirrhosis between 1979 and 1983. The table also includes three low risk jobs. The average job had a rate of 100,

Table 6.2 Liver cirrhosis mortality amongst British males in different occupations (1979–80, 1982–83)

Occupational group	Mortality rate
Average occupation	100
Publicans	1,017
Deck, engine room hands, bargemen, lightermen, boatmen	873
Barmen	612
Deck, engineering and radio officers and pilots, ship	417
Electrical engineers (so described)	387
Hotel and residential club managers	342
Innkeepers	315
Fishermen	296
Chefs, cooks	265
Restaurateurs	263
Authors, writers, journalists	261
Drivers' mates	225
Winders, reelers	202
Other domestic and school helpers	141
Garage proprietors	140
Medical practitioners	115
Farm workers	45
Printing machine minders and assistants	32
Managers in building and contracting	22

Source: Office of Population Censuses and Surveys (Personal Communication) (1986)

so each of the sixteen 'high risk' occupations included in Table 6.2 had rates of between 1.1 and 10.2 times the average. Research has shown that Scottish male doctors and trawlermen are three times more likely than comparable workers to be diagnosed as alcohol dependent. Male British doctors who died during the periods 1979–80 and 1982–83 and who were aged 55–64 had a liver cirrhosis death rate over *twice* the occupational average. In addition, brewery and distillery workers have been found to drink more heavily and develop more alcohol problems than workers in 'drier' jobs. As shown on Table 6.2 a varied group of occupations have high rates of liver cirrhosis mortality. These include the drink trade, fishing and other sea-faring jobs, journalism and catering. It is difficult to identify common factors which might link such different types of employment. The following eight factors are those most often suggested to explain why some jobs do have such a high rate of alcohol problem:

1 Availability of alcohol at work (e.g. drink trade).
2 Social pressure to drink at work (e.g. servicemen, seamen).
3 Separation from normal social or sexual relationships (e.g. servicemen, seamen, commercial travellers).
4 Freedom from supervision (e.g. executives, doctors, lawyers).
5 Very high or very low income levels (e.g. professionals, the unemployed or unskilled workers).
6 Collusion by colleagues (fear of dismissal or exploiting a colleague's incapacity).
7 Strains and stresses, e.g. danger (seamen, servicemen); responsibility (doctors, lawyers, executives); job insecurity (actors); boredom, etc.
8 Recruitment of 'unusual people' predisposed to drink heavily (e.g. Merchant Navy).

Sex differences

As noted in Chapter 5, males universally drink much more than females. Even so, the differences between the drinking habits of the sexes is changing steadily. During the past two decades there has been a steady increase in recorded levels of alcohol problems among women. Alcoholics Anonymous have reported that while in 1964 only one in five of their members was female, now a third of them are. Similarly all types of agencies providing help for alcohol problems have reported a steady, dramatic and disproportionate increase in the numbers of women consulting them. This change appears to have been slightly slower in Scotland than in England and Wales. Even so, most agencies now report that at least a quarter or a third of their clients are women. The Merseyside, Cheshire and Lancashire Council on Alcoholism has noted that among their clients under the age of thirty, there were equal numbers of males and females. A general review of trends in British alcohol problems conducted by Duffy and Plant (1986) concluded that the rate of increase of alcohol problems amongst women (and their recent decline) was generally parallel to trends amongst males.

Evidence from Britain and from other Western countries shows that women with alcohol problems drink much less than their male counterparts, often only a third or half as much. In spite of this, females generally report experiencing the same range of harmful consequences as do males. It appears that female problem drinkers are in fact more socially isolated, more often divorced, have experienced more childhood disruption and are in poorer general health than males. Possibly husbands are less willing or able to tolerate and support a heavily drinking wife than is the case if the wife is expected to help or accept a heavily drinking husband.

Females are more vulnerable to liver disease than are males. In addition they are less likely to recover even if they cut down or cease their drinking. This difference is partly attributable to the lower average body weight of females. It is also due to females' greater physical vulnerability to the effect of alcohol. As shown in Table 6.3, women in Britain have a liver cirrhosis rate that is disproportionately high in relation to their alcohol consumption.

Women are generally no younger than males when they first contact agencies for help with alcohol problems. In spite of this women frequently report that they began excessive drinking later in life and that they experienced alcohol problems relatively soon thereafter. Women seem less likely than men to become problem drinkers for purely casual social reasons, but

Table 6.3   *Rates of liver cirrhosis mortality in twenty five countries (1983)*

Country	Males	Females	Total
Australia**	10.7	4.4	7.6
Austria**	43.8	18.0	30.2
Bulgaria**	20.4	7.6	13.9
Canada**	13.0	6.4	9.7
Czechoslovakia	29.8	11.2	20.3
Finland	9.7	4.5	7.0
France (1981)**	39.5	16.2	27.6
Germany, West**	34.6	16.4	25.1
Hungary**	55.7	23.8	39.2
Ireland (1981)	3.5	2.9	3.2
Israel**	5.9	4.6	5.3
Italy (1980)	49.1	20.1	34.3
Japan**	20.3	8.0	14.1
Luxembourg**	27.6	13.2	20.2
Netherlands**	6.7	3.9	5.3
New Zealand	4.7	2.8	3.8
Norway	7.6	4.1	5.8
Panama**	5.6	1.9	3.8
Poland**	13.2	7.5	10.3
Portugal (1982)**	44.6	16.6	30.1
Sweden (1982)	12.6	5.0	8.7
Switzerland	18.6	6.5	12.4
UK – England and Wales (1982)**	4.7	4.0	4.3
– Scotland**	9.8	7.0	8.4
USA (1982)**	15.9	8.2	12.0

Rates are calculated per 100,000 population
** Chronic liver disease and cirrhosis
Source: World Health Organisation 1984, 1985

seem especially likely to develop alcohol problems in reaction to specific events, such as bereavement or divorce, or because their role in life changes. Sometimes women develop alcohol problems when their family grows up and 'leaves the nest'. Women problem drinkers often feel more guilty about their drinking than do their male counterparts.

It has been suggested that heavy drinking by pregnant women may cause foetal damage. This 'foetal alcohol syndrome' appears to be rare but has recently been revived as a cause for concern. This may reflect the recent increase in alcohol consumption by women, especially by those of child-bearing age. As noted in Chapter 2 evidence suggests that although maternal alcohol consumption is associated with birth abnormalities so too are a host of other factors. The potential dangers of alcohol consumption during pregnancy have been greatly exaggerated. Heavy drinking may be harmful and should be avoided. Even so there is no evidence that moderate drinking is harmful.

Although female drinking habits are changing there persists a greater stigma of alcohol misuse by females than by males. In consequence women with alcohol problems first may be less likely to seek help for their difficulties than would males. Secondly, females with alcohol problems are often regarded by their families, the community, therapists and fellow clients or patients in a less sympathetic manner than are comparable males.

National differences

There are no grounds for complacency about the alarming growth of alcohol problems in Britain. Even so, it is worth placing British experience in an international context. As noted in Chapter 5, the general level of alcohol consumption in the UK is much lower than that in most other western countries. This is reflected by the fact that the rate of liver cirrhosis deaths in the UK is also very much lower than in many other countries. This is shown in Table 6.3.

Liver cirrhosis is only one form of alcohol problem. There is no doubt that the overwhelming majority of alcohol problems are *social* rather than *physical* ones. Treatment agencies and laws vary greatly, even within Britain. It is therefore not very useful to attempt to draw too many conclusions about how the overall level of alcohol problems in Britain compares with that elsewhere. Even so, it is generally accepted by researchers that the countries with the highest rates of alcohol problems are those such as France, where levels of alcohol consumption are especially high. It is also clear from a considerable body of evidence that the rates of alcohol problems, such as liver cirrhosis deaths, drunkenness and drunken driving convictions and psychiatric hospital admissions for alcohol dependence are clearly related to the general level of alcohol consumption. Such rates rose with alcohol consumption during the 1960s and 1970s. They have declined as alcohol consumption in the United Kingdom has fallen since 1979. Alcohol problems, as noted by Peck (1982), are influenced by a wide variety of social, psychological and biological factors so that some people and some social groups are more vulnerable than others to experiencing alcohol-related problems. Even so it is emphasised that *anybody* who drinks a lot runs the risk of experiencing adverse consequences.

Tobacco-related harm

Smokers do not live as long as non-smokers do. The Royal College of Physicians in their report, *Health or Smoking?* (1983) estimated that 100,000 people each year were dying prematurely of tobacco-related diseases in the United Kingdom. They emphasised the scale of this carnage thus:

> 'Among 1,000 young male adults in England and Wales who smoke cigarettes, on average about:
> 1 will be murdered
> 8 will be killed on the roads
> 250 will be killed before their time by tobacco'. (Royal College of Physicians 1983: 2)

Smoking now causes approximately 90% of all lung cancer deaths in Britain, together with over a third of all other British cancer deaths.

Cigarette smoking is very likely to produce dependence. Tobacco dependence is the most widespread form of drug dependence in the world. As stated by Russell (1974): 'It is probably the most addictive and dependence-producing form of object-specific self-administered gratification known to man.' The great majority of smokers do not restrict themselves to only occasional use of tobacco and most will continue to smoke.

The health risks of smoking are well documented and appalling. Smokers place much greater demands on the health services than do non-smokers. Apart from reducing their life expectancy, smokers are also especially likely to experience prolonged ill-health. As the Royal College of Physicians noted in their 1977 Report:

> 'Patients who ultimately die from chronic bronchitis or emphysema usually endure about ten years of distressing breathlessness before they die. Cigarette smokers are also more liable than non-smokers to attacks of acute bronchitis, and other chest illnesses. In Britain as many as fifty million working days may be lost in industry every year as a consequence of cigarette smoking.'

Smokers are *twice* as likely as non-smokers to die before the age of sixty-five. Research into the smoking habits of British doctors indicated that a person who smokes twenty cigarettes each day will reduce his or her lifespan by about five years. The World Health Organisation (1979) has suggested that smoking accounts for a high proportion of male deaths from lung cancer (90%), bronchitis (75%) and ischaemic heart disease (25%). These percentages are probably rather lower for females. As the World Health Organisation has noted: 'The strongest evidence that cigarette smoking is responsible for excess mortality is the reduction that occurs after cessation of smoking.'

Recent trends

Between 1972 and 1978, as noted in the previous chapter, the decline in cigarette smoking was more marked in males than in females. Consistent with these relative changes, lung cancer deaths among women aged forty-five and above have increased steeply. Table 6.4 depicts the age distribution of males and females dying of tobacco-related illnesses in the United Kingdom during 1974. As shown, 9% of those in this category were aged only thirty-five to forty-four.

Bronchitis deaths have declined for both sexes. This is probably due to improved treatment and restrictions on air pollution. Table 6.4 is limited to those aged thirty-five to sixty-four since among those aged sixty-five and above it seems that only a small proportion of deaths are attributable to smoking. Old age and other causes obviously become much more important.

Regional variations

The Office of Population Censuses and Surveys has reviewed regional variations in deaths from tobacco-related diseases in England and Wales 1970–2. This analysis showed that the rates of lung cancer deaths were

Table 6.4 *Age distribution of those aged thirty-five to sixty-four dying of tobacco-related diseases (United Kingdom) (1977)*

Age	Males N	Males %	Females N	Females %	Total N	Total %
35–44	7,448	8	5,038	9	12,486	9
45–54	25,864	28	15,972	29	41,836	28
55–64	59,703	64	34,342	62	94,045	63
Total	93,015	100%	55,352	100%	148,367	100%

Percentages are rounded off to the nearest whole number
Source: Royal College of Physicians (1977)

highest in the North and North West of England. The rates of ischaemic heart disease deaths were also high in Northern England and North Wales, but were highest in South Wales. Deaths due to bronchitis, emphysema and asthma were highest in North and North West England and in South Wales. The Scottish rates of lung cancer are higher than those in England and Wales, both for males and for females. The corresponding rates in Northern Ireland are lower than elsewhere in the United Kingdom as shown in Table 6.6 on p. 101.

Occupational variations

Consistent with the evidence described above that some occupations have especially high rates of alcohol problems, some also have especially high rates of tobacco related mortality. The lung cancer death rates of fifteen selected occupational groups of men in Britain during the period 1979–80 and 1982–83 are shown in Table 6.5.

Table 6.5 *Mortality from malignant neoplasm of trachea, bronchus and lung amongst British men in different occupations (1979–80, 1982–83)*

Occupation	Mortality Rates
Average occupation	100
Labourers and unskilled workers NEC – coalminers	204
Metal plate workers, shipwrights, riveters	200
Publicans	167
Machine tool operators	163
Sheet metal workers	147
Drivers of road goods vehicles	146
Welders	146
Innkeepers	143
Bricklayers, tilesetters	137
Builders (so described)	131
Face-trained coalmining workers	116
Clerks of work	75
Chartered and certified accountants	46
Medical practitioners	25
University academic staff	21

Source: Office of Population Censuses and Surveys (Personal Communication) (1986)

The highest rates shown in Table 6.5 are not as dramatically high as those for liver cirrhosis depicted in Table 6.2. Nevertheless, as the preceding table shows, coalminers are roughly ten times as likely as university teachers to die of lung cancer. Publicans and innkeepers are roughly seven times as likely to die of lung cancer as doctors. High rates of tobacco related diseases are now especially commonplace amongst manual workers. It is also notable that publicans and innkeepers, in a very distinctive occupational setting, have high rates of alcohol and tobacco related deaths.

Surveys have shown that there is a clear relationship between smoking habits and lung cancer rates for men in specific occupational groups. Smoking greatly increases health risks even in jobs such as coal mining, in which there are other obvious causes of lung cancer and other tobacco-related diseases. The World Health Organisation (1979) commented on the influence of occupation thus:

'The difference in health between smokers and non-smokers may be substantially aggravated by occupation. The combined effects of smoking and other environmental hazards, mainly occupational in nature, have been extensively studied during the past few years . . .

Many studies of workers in the mechanical, chemical, ceramics, foundry, corn-mill, mining, tyre cutting, asbestos, construction, cement, rubber, cork and other industries have shown a higher incidence of respiratory diseases among smokers than among non-smokers exposed to the same occupational hazards. Smokers present a high prevalence of morning cough, and production of phlegm and dyspnoea, chronic bronchitis and other chronic non-specific bronchopulmonary diseases are more frequent among them . . . smoking habits potentiate the effects of some carcinogens (cancer causing substances) such as arsenic, nickel . . . and asbestos . . .

Specific occupational groups such as uranium miners, workers in the chromium, nickel and asbestos industries, painters and carpenters have an increased risk of lung cancer, and this risk is considerably augmented if the individual also smokes cigarettes . . . Investigations to identify ischaemic heart disease risks in airline pilots showed a clear-cut dose-response relationship between smoking and various pathological findings. A forty-five-year-old male pilot who smokes twenty cigarettes a day has a risk of sudden death 2.8 times greater than that of a non-smoking pilot, irrespective of other risk factors.'

It has been frequently noted that (predominantly male) doctors in Britain have drastically reduced their smoking in contrast to (predominantly female) nurses who appear often to smoke heavily. British doctors, more than any other occupational group, have been bombarded with scientific evidence that smoking is a potentially lethal pursuit. Between 1951 and 1971 cigarette consumption by doctors aged thirty-five to fifty-nine fell from 10.5 to 3.5 per day. This decline was accompanied by a 22% fall in the death rate of doctors in this age group. Older doctors (many of whom remained confirmed pipe smokers) originally had a much lower level of cigarette consumption than their younger counterparts. Their cigarette consumption *rose* during this period as pipe smokers died and were replaced by cigarette smokers.

Research has shown that while many medical students smoke, they are much more aware of the inherent health risks associated with this practice than are student nurses. It is also evident that absenteeism and ill-health are much more prevalent among nurses who smoke than among those who do not. Similar evidence is available showing that workers who smoke are generally less healthy and miss more work than non-smokers.

Sex differences

As noted in Chapter 5, female smokers generally consume fewer cigarettes per week than males. In addition males have traditionally been more likely to smoke than females although as also noted in the previous chapter, this is no longer the case in Britain. Even so, males are universally far more likely than females to die of lung cancer as a result of their (originally) high tobacco consumption. This disparity is shown in Table 6.6. The British lung cancer death rate for males in 1975 was roughly five times greater than that for females. As stated in Chapter 2, tobacco smoking by pregnant women is associated with reduced birth weights in offspring. Mothers who smoke twenty cigarettes daily produce babies roughly ¾ lb lighter than those of non-smoking mothers. In addition there is evidence that even *fathers'* cigarette smoke, if inhaled by a pregnant mother, sometimes causes similar reductions in birth weight. Smoking also appears to increase the risks of congenital malformations in children whose mothers smoke while pregnant. Spontaneous abortions, stillbirths and deaths during labour or soon after birth are also commoner among mothers who smoke. In addition there is evidence that smoking is especially dangerous to females using oral contraceptives and that smoking leads to an earlier menopause.

National differences

Levels of tobacco-related diseases vary enormously between different countries. Table 6.6 shows rates of death per 100,000 population due to lung cancer in twenty four countries during 1955 and 1975. As the table shows, such rates universally rose considerably during this period reflecting a steady post-war rise in cigarette smoking.

As Table 6.6 indicates, the United Kingdom has an exceptionally high rate of lung cancer mortality. It is generally agreed to be the highest in the world. Between 1955 and 1975, as Table 6.6 shows, the rate of lung cancer mortality among males in England and Wales increased by roughly 38%. The

Table 6.6. *Rates* of lung cancer mortality in twenty four countries (1955–75)*

	Sex	1955	1975
Austria	M	41.7	50.7
	F	5.0	6.7
Australia	M	20.2	46.0
	F	2.9	7.0
Belgium	M	26.6	67.3
	F	3.7	5.7
Czechoslovakia	M	33.8	65.2†
	F	5.6	5.4†
Canada	M	20.0	46.1†
	F	4.1	8.8†
Denmark	M	20.9	45.7
	F	4.5	10.7
Finland	M	47.0	64.1†
	F	4.5	4.2†
France	M	16.0	35.1†
	F	3.3	3.5†
Hungary	M	20.3	47.1
	F	5.3	8.0
Irish Republic	M	18.6	44.2
	F	5.4	13.8
Italy	M	14.3	41.8†
	F	3.3	5.1†
Netherlands	M	30.0	71.5
	F	2.8	4.2
New Zealand	M	25.6	48.7
	F	3.0	10.6
Norway	M	7.8	22.3
	F	2.7	4.5
Portugal	M	7.6	15.1
	F	2.0	3.3
Spain	M	–	26.6†
	F	–	4.2†
Sweden	M	10.8	23.6
	F	5.1	6.0
Switzerland	M	26.9	47.6
	F	2.9	4.4
United Kingdom –	M	51.7	71.8
England and Wales	F	6.6	14.6

Table 6.6. continued

	Sex	1955	1975
United Kingdom – Scotland	M	50.0	82.7
	F	7.4	15.8
United Kingdom – N. Ireland	M	30.1	52.6
	F	4.0	11.7
USA	M	24.2	51.0
	F	4.0	12.5
West Germany	M	25.6	47.3
	F	4.1	5.1
Yugoslavia	M	–	32.6
	F	–	5.5

* Rates are age standardised per 100,000 total population
† Figures relate to 1974
Source: World Health Organisation 1979

corresponding increase among females was roughly 120%. Similarly in Scotland and Northern Ireland, female rates increased disproportionately and dramatically, by 113% and 190% respectively. The corresponding male rates of increase were 65% (Scotland) and 74% (Northern Ireland). While similar rates of increase have been evident almost universally, the very high level of lung cancer mortality in the United Kingdom, especially in Scotland, England and Wales, is a major cause for concern.

Which smoking is worst?

All smokers run much greater health risks than non-smokers. Even so, it is clear that cigarette smoking, which is by far the most popular form of tobacco use, is far more dangerous than either pipe or cigar smoking. This is probably attributable to the fact that cigarette smokers are especially likely to inhale tobacco products into their lungs. This practice greatly increases the risks to the smoker's health. Filter tip cigarettes are 'safer' than the non-filter type and low tar cigarettes are 'safer' than higher tar cigarettes. It must be emphasised that this 'safety' is only a relative one. All tobacco smoking involves health risks. The overall risk depends upon the amounts smoked, the amounts inhaled and the age of starting to smoke. The younger one starts, the longer one is exposed to health risks.

'Passive smoking'

Smoking gets up other people's noses. This is, obviously, obnoxious. There is only limited evidence that 'passive' smoking causes lung cancer. Even so, it has been established that breathing other people's cigarette smoke does impair lung function. The health of infants is clearly harmed if they are subjected to a smoky atmosphere at home. If both parents smoke twenty or more cigarettes a day their offspring run a doubled risk of suffering from serious respiratory conditions during the first year of life.

Non-smokers commonly report irritation of the nose, eyes and throat and sometimes nausea and headaches due to inhaling smoke from other people's cigarettes. These effects are worst in confined, poorly ventilated spaces. People with respiratory problems (such as asthma) may be more seriously harmed by involuntary inhalation of cigarette smoke. One effect of breathing in other people's smoke is that carbon monoxide levels may be increased and thereby impede perceptions and abilities to react quickly or perform precise tasks such as driving. Smoking in the company of non-smokers is not a private affair.

Drug offences

During the past decade police forces throughout the United Kingdom have established drug squads of officers whose special responsibility is to enforce the drug control laws. In consequence the increased level of police activity in this field has led to a steady increase in the numbers of drug offenders detected and brought to court. The number of drug seizures have also greatly increased. It must be emphasised that Home Office statistics of drug seizures and offences *do not* in themselves serve as an indication of the extent of drug use in the community. Such figures reflect many other factors including police policies, methods of detection and the conspicuousness or ineptitude of drug users and traffickers.

Seizures of drugs

It is probable that HM Customs and Excise Officers, the police and other officials only manage to seize a small proportion of all drugs illegally imported or distributed. Even so, large quantities of drugs have been seized and some notable successes have been recorded in detecting large-scale illicit drug trafficking especially in 1980. Over 90% of all seizures involve cannabis in some form and this is reflected by the fact that most people convicted under the *Misuse of Drugs Act* (1971) are charged with cannabis offences. The scale of drug seizures during the period 1974–84 is shown in Table 6.7.

Table 6.7 provides only an indication of the quantities of drugs seized during the period 1973–84. Individual seizures vary enormously. For example, during 1977 relatively few LSD seizures were recorded, yet the quantity impounded was considerable due to the success of 'Operation Julie' in which roughly 15,000,000 doses were seized. Other very large-scale

Table 6.7 Seizures of controlled drugs by drug type[1]

Drug type	1974	1975	1976	1977	1978	1979	1980	1981	1982	1983	1984
Class 'A' drugs											
Cocaine	215	218	230	204	257	348	445	503	389	684	889
Dextromoramide	50	60	55	61	56	79	86	80	77	51	75
Dipipanone	150	192	158	241	283	349	259	370	428	292	162
Heroin	310	236	347	270	346	600	697	819	985	1,940	2,995
Methadone	302	260	252	212	235	292	328	402	360	412	503
Morphine	320	300	263	347	289	319	294	243	191	156	158
Opium	128	182	124	149	121	299	218	137	105	88	73
Pethidine	168	162	166	173	157	169	172	135	110	78	75
LSD	601	626	434	202	289	216	268	384	464	518	629
Other class 'A' drugs	213	156	144	230	138	100	113	119	145	96	119
All class 'A' drugs	1,835	1,777	1,700	1,523	1,622	2,087	2,196	2,513	2,670	3,763	4,994

Drug type	1974	1975	1976	1977	1978	1979	1980	1981	1982	1983	1984
Class 'B' drugs											
Cannabis	3,893	3,835	3,912	3,238	3,986	5,564	8,830	8,500	8,775	8,929	9,730
Cannabis plants	325	436	628	872	820	1,324	2,351	1,787	1,708	1,296	1,806
Cannabis resin	5,124	4,969	6,108	8,080	8,247	8,826	6,964	8,911	10,679	13,976	13,978
Cannabis liquid	83	190	137	126	88	191	223	254	284	313	224
Amphetamine Dexamphetamine Levamphetamine	857	915	1,255	960	586	632	666	1,076	1,645	2,329	2,756
Methylamphetamine	48	211	195	434	89	119	78	44	10	8	94
Other Class 'B' drugs	373	283	194	222	221	289	217	243	246	192	114
All class 'B' drugs	9,435	9,454	10,719	12,065	12,416	14,700	16,228	17,953	20,124	23,952[2]	25,149
Class 'C' drugs											
Methaqualone	574	408	300	329	298	336	296	143	58	32	28
Other class 'C' drugs	13	13	11	10	6	12	19	11	4	6	98
All class 'C' drugs	582	411	306	334	300	344	308	152	62	38	125
All controlled drugs	10,817	10,648	11,800	13,006	13,454	16,056	17,617	19,428	21,636	26,216	28,560

[1] As the same seizure can involve more than one drug type, rows cannot be added together to produce sub-totals or totals.
[2] Revised figure.

seizures have been recorded, notably 'Operation Cyril' during which 4,295 kilograms of cannabis (roughly 4.2 tons) were intercepted in only two seizures during 1979.

Drug offences

There has been a steady increase in the number of drug offences recorded by the Home Office. In 1945 only four cannabis offences were recorded, together with 200 for opium and twenty for manufactured drugs. Since that date the number of persons convicted annually for cannabis offences has increased to more than 18,000 and in 1985 the total number of people cautioned or convicted of drug offences was 26,596. Convictions for drug offences during the period 1979–84 are shown in Table 6.8.

As Table 6.8 shows, the great majority of those convicted, roughly 80%, are found guilty of offences related to cannabis. During the period 1979–84 the majority of offenders (at least 85% in any single year) were convicted of *possessing* controlled drugs. Even so, during this period the proportion of offences of other types, such as illegal importing, exporting of drugs and cultivating cannabis plants, increased slightly.

By far the largest group of drug offenders (71% in 1984) are people convicted of possessing cannabis. It is clear that by any criterion the great

Table 6.8 *Persons* found guilty of drug offences (1979–1984)*

Type of drug	1979	1980	1981	1982	1983	1984
Cocaine	330	475	565	425	563	696
Heroin	517	749	806	963	1,489	2,404
Methadone	296	362	445	402	378	406
Dipipanone (Diconal)	451	439	496	564	367	251
LSD	203	245	344	460	440	536
Cannabis	12,156	14,690	15,153	16,958	18,845	18,515
Amphetamines	755	821	1,065	1,500	1,981	2,449
Other Drugs	1,151	1,281	1,130	945	930	955
All Drugs	14,054	16,919	17,667	19,833	22,158	22,882

* As the same person may be found guilty of offences involving more than one drug, rows cannot be added together to produce totals.

Source: Home Office 1985

majority of individuals convicted of drug offences are not large-scale commercial dealers. Most are convicted of possessing amounts of drugs consistent with their own personal usage. The extent of large-scale criminal involvement in illegal drug supply is unclear, although it is certain that such involvement has greatly increased during recent years.

Some people are clearly prepared to risk the legal consequences by trafficking in large amounts of controlled drugs, as demonstrated by the huge seizures obtained by operations 'Julie' and 'Cyril'. In addition, as during alcohol prohibition in America, such trafficking sometimes leads to violence. During recent years several people have been murdered in drug-related crimes in the United Kingdom.

General characteristics of drug offenders

The great majority of those cautioned or convicted drug offenders are young males. In 1984 77% were under the age of thirty and the average age of such offenders was twenty-six and 88% were males.

Sentencing policies

Roughly 80% of those sentenced for drug offences receive a non-custodial punishment such as a fine. Juveniles (those aged under seventeen) are especially unlikely to receive a custodial sentence such as imprisonment or a suspended sentence. As noted above, most drug offences involve possessing cannabis. More than half of those convicted of the illegal supply, production, export and import of drugs are given a custodial sentence. Clearly the courts take a much more serious view of 'drug pushing' than of drug possession. In 1984 67% of those convicted of drug trafficking received custodial sentences.

Recorded addicts

The Home Office records individuals notified by doctors as being dependent upon and *currently* receiving prescriptions of opiates and cocaine. Such notifications are received from drug treatment centres, prisons and from general practitioners. As noted in the previous chapter, it is probable that only a minority of all those using opiates are included in Home Office records. There is certainly a flourishing black market in such drugs, the extent of which can only be guessed. A 5% sample postal survey of general practitioners in England and Wales indicated that the annual number of new 'addicts' was between 30,000 and 44,000 (Glanz and Taylor 1986). As shown in Table 6.9, there was a steady rise in the number of people recorded as 'narcotic drug addicts' since 1970. This has gained momentum since 1978. In 1981 the increase, 36%, was particularly marked.

Table 6.9 *Narcotic drug addicts known to the Home Office**
(1970–1984)

Year	Males	Females	Total	Change Over Previous Years
1970	1,051	375	1,426	–
1971	1,133	416	1,549	+ 9%
1972	1,195	421	1,616	+ 4%
1973	1,370	446	1,816	+ 12%
1974	1,458	509	1,967	+ 8%
1975	1,438	511	1,949	− 1%
1976	1,387	487	1,874	− 4%
1977	1,466	550	2,016	+ 6%
1978	1,703	699	2,402	+ 19%
1979	1,892	774	2,666	+ 11%
1980	2,009	837	2,846	+ 7%
1981	2,732	1,112	3,844	+ 36%
1982	3,124	1,247	4,371	+ 14%
1983	3,601	1,478	5,079	+ 16%
1984	4,133	1,736	5,869	+ 15%

* At 31 December each year.
† Figures rounded to nearest %
Source: Home Office 1979–1985

Most notified 'drug addicts' are young. The age distribution of those recorded in 1984 is shown in Table 6.10.

The Home Office records are by no means a complete measure of dependence upon notifiable drugs. They exclude addicts whom doctors have failed to notify. In addition it has been suggested that individuals dependent upon dipipanone (Diconal) are especially unlikely to be recorded as such. Also, the Home Office figures do not refer to those who have discontinued recorded opiate use, even if only temporarily. Throughout the 1970s roughly two-thirds of recorded addicts were being prescribed methadone alone. In 1984 85% of addicts received only methadone, compared with only 1.6% who received only heroin. The distribution of types of drugs prescribed during 1984 is shown in Table 6.11.

General characteristics of drugtakers attending treatment agencies

Many young drugtakers contact counselling, helping and treatment agencies without necessarily using opiates or cocaine or being dependent on drugs.

Table 6.10 *Age distribution of narcotic drug addicts known to the Home Office at 31 December 1984.*

Age	Males	Females
Under 21	203	95
21 and under 25	594	318
25 and under 30	961	501
30 and under 35	1,323	455
35 and under 50	857	238
50 and over	133	96
Not recorded	62	33
Total	4,133	1,736
Average age	31.2	30.8

Source: Home Office 1985

Table 6.11 *Types of drugs prescribed to notified addicts during 1984*

Drug	Number of Persons
Methadone alone	5,010
Methadone and heroin	75
Methadone, heroin and other drugs	2
Methadone and other drugs but not heroin	73
Heroin alone	97
Heroin and other drugs but not methadone	8
Morphine alone	33
Pethidine alone	41
Dextromoamide alone	109
Dipipanone (Diconal) alone	386
Cocaine alone	3
Other drugs alone	24
Other drug combination	8
Total	5,869

Source: Home Office 1985

The motivation leading to such help seeking is very varied. Some people are drawn by a wish to obtain drugs. Others attend because they are on a court charge or have been in trouble with the police. Sometimes individuals with a drug-related court appearance hanging over them hope a psychiatric or social work report may help to exonerate them or at least will minimise penalties if convicted. Very many young people who contact helping agencies are motivated by social pressure (for example by parents) or because of a fright such as an overdose or a bad LSD trip. All studies confirm that most, probably around three-quarters, of drugtakers known to clinics are males. In addition, all social classes are represented, even though a disproportionate number of young clinic attenders come from manual backgrounds. A very high proportion are either unemployed or have extremely poor work records, often drifting from one unskilled job to the next.

One of the most detailed British studies of opiate users at clinics was carried out by Stimson and Oppenheimer (1982). This research is referred to in Chapter 7 because it not only collected information about clinic offenders, but followed up their progress ten years later. This study related to 111 heroin users comprising a representative sample of those in London clinics. Nearly three-quarters were males and the average age of these 111 people was twenty-five years. The majority, 76%, were born in England and Wales, 4% were Scottish and 12% were born in Northern Ireland or Eire. Stimson's study confirmed that by no means all opiate dependants are drawn from the lowest social class backgrounds, even if these are particularly highly represented. Some of those who seek help from clinics in relation to their drugtaking come from professional family backgrounds and are hardly 'deprived' in a material sense.

There is a consensus from available evidence that most of those attending drug treatment clinics are young, unmarried and male. The percentage of females has been noted in some areas to be increasing and as noted above this applies to those recorded as opiate dependants. There is little doubt that individuals seeking help from drug treatment clinics are a highly disturbed group. It has been widely noted that drug troubles are often combined with all manner of other difficulties, animosity to (and by) parents, unemployment, conflict with the law, homelessness, parasuicide and a considerable amount of social and psychological turmoil. Even so, drugtakers are not unique in this respect and several studies have suggested that other groups of 'deviant' young people have equally colourful biographies.

Those attending drug clinics, even those recorded as opiate dependants, are an extremely varied group. Stimson (1973) suggested that the drug users in his study could be sub-divided into four different groups.

1 The Stables
These tend to use drugs alone and are all in full or part-time employment. Their drug use is not a social activity. They are not assimilated into the

'counter-culture' of the drug scene. Such drug users conceal their drug use from others and continue to have 'normal' relationships with family and colleagues.

2 The Junkies
These are socially disorganised, 'deviant' individuals whose lifestyles are bizarre and whose drug use is indiscriminate. They are deeply involved with the drug scene, and often indulge in crime to buy drugs, often on the black market.

3 The Two-worlders
These combine a high level of employment with considerable criminal activity and involvement with the drug scene. They are part of both the 'workaday world' and of the drug scene.

4 The Loners
These share the junkie's poor work record but do not depend upon crime. They rely upon Social Security and other non-criminal sources of income. They are much less involved with other drug users than are the junkies and two-worlders.

Types of drugs used

A very high proportion of young drug clinic attenders report that not only are they heavy users of alcohol and tobacco but that they have extremely catholic tastes in relation to other drugs. Polydrug use, experimentation with a wide range of legal and illegal substances, has been cited in the previous chapter on general patterns of drug use. Those who seek help from drug counselling and treatment agencies are especially likely to be deeply involved in the lifestyles of 'the drug scene' and are also likely to report using a wide range of drugs. It is evident that many young people, deeply involved with drugtaking, are prepared to use virtually any substance and that most do not use opiates or other drugs often enough to become physically dependent upon them. Stimson reported that London heroin users had also used cannabis (100%), opiates other than heroin (97%), tranquillisers (81%), cocaine (94%), psychedelics (65%), sedatives and hypnotics (95%), amphetamine, amphetamine/barbiturate mixtures and other stimulants (98%). Similarly, a review by the author concluded that polydrug use was the norm among seventy-two young drugtakers attending the Royal Edinburgh Hospital. The range of substances reportedly used by the latter individuals is shown in Table 6.12.

Very many drugtakers attending clinics have conspicuous alcohol problems. Some are 'officially labelled' as alcohol dependants rather than as 'drug dependants'. It is clear that just as in more general terms, alcohol and tobacco are often used as well as illegal drugs, so some of those using illegal drugs excessively or harmfully will often be unusually heavy users of alcohol and tobacco as well as of prescribed drugs such as tranquillisers.

Table 6.12 *Drugs ever taken 'for kicks' by seventy-two Scottish hospital attenders*

Drug	N
Cannabis	51
Amphetamines	38
LSD	34
Heroin	29
Barbiturates	27
Mandrax	25
Morphine	22
Methadone	13
Opium	9
Mescalin	9
Tuinal	7
Cocaine	5
Valium	5
Omnopon	3
Cough linctuses	3
Methedrine	3
Inhalers	2
Librium	2
Diconal	1
Preludin	1
Palfrium	1
Demerol	1
Largactil	1
Solvents/glues	1

Drug overdoses

Drug overdoses have been described as one of the great modern epidemics. It was once widely assumed that people who survived taking deliberate overdoses of drugs were unsuccessful suicides. The phrase 'attempted suicide' is still widely applied to such events. Researchers have pointed out for some years that the types of people who successfully commit suicide differ in some important and quite definite ways from those whose overdoses or other comparable acts do not result in death. It is now clear that most 'attempted suicides' are not intended to be fatal. For this reason recent writings on the subject have suggested that other terms such as 'self-poisoning' are more accurate descriptions of this type of behaviour. Moreover it is now generally accepted by most researchers in the field that most 'accidental' self-poisoning by either gas or drugs is seldom inadvertent.

Some researchers favour the use of the term *parasuicide* to indicate behaviour that is in certain respects related to suicide but not motivated by a wish to die. *Parasuicide* is defined in the following terms:

'Parasuicide is a non-fatal act in which an individual deliberately causes self-injury or ingests a substance in excess of any prescribed or generally recognised therapeutic dosage' (Kreitman 1977).

This definition has generally been applied to exclude those under the influence of alcohol alone, but does cover those who have overdosed with other psychoactive drugs either alone or in combination with alcohol. Overdoses and other adverse reactions to drugs taken illegally or 'for kicks' are also included in this definition.

Drug overdoses account for over 90% of deliberate self-injuries in Britain. Parasuicide has increased steadily in most Western countries since the 1960s, although during the last few years this increase has levelled off, or even begun to decrease in some areas. There are no national figures available, but research in centres such as Bristol, Edinburgh, London, Oxford, Sheffield and Southampton has been reviewed (Dyer 1980). This review emphasised that parasuicide placed a major burden on the medical services of Britain. A Glasgow study indicated that parasuicides constituted 15% of all medical admissions to the Western Infirmary in that city. Dyer calculated that roughly 10% of all admissions to Edinburgh hospitals are parasuicides and noted that similar conclusions have been drawn in other areas. It is further evident that parasuicides constitute between 20–30% of medical emergencies in British hospitals. There is no doubt that parasuicide places a huge burden on hospital emergency departments, psychiatric hospitals and social work services.

Those most likely to indulge in parasuicide are young. The peak ages for males and females are twenty to twenty-four and fifteen to nineteen respectively. Parasuicides have increased steadily during the past fifteen years in contrast to the suicide rate which has *declined* slightly. As Dyer has noted, there are further differences between these two phenomena:

'Parasuicide is at least 10–20 times as common as suicide. The age/sex distribution is different; while the incidence of parasuicide is greater in females and in younger people, that of suicide is greater in males and older people.'

Even so, there does exist a clear relationship between parasuicide and suicide. This has, again, been succinctly summarised by Dyer:

'The risk of suicide is much greater in those with a history of parasuicide than in the general population. While it is a small proportion who go on to kill themselves, they form nearly half of all suicides.'

The pattern of substances used in parasuicide (and suicide) has changed considerably during recent years. Once gassing was a commonplace method of committing suicide. The introduction of non-toxic natural gas has been identified as a major factor in the recent decline in suicides. The increased availability of drugs has been reflected in the increased use of such substances for the purposes of both suicide and, more commonly, parasuicide. The types of drugs used in these ways have reflected prescribing patterns. A review of admissions to Edinburgh's Regional Poisoning Treatment Centre showed that between 1967 and 1976 the annual number of admissions more than doubled. In addition the proportion of admissions related to barbiturates and methaqualone (Mandrax) declined markedly while those associated with benzodiazepines, especially Valium, and tricyclic antidepressants increased. An important effect of the increased 'popularity' of 'safer' drugs in parasuicide was that fewer patients were admitted unconscious. The authors also noted that during the period covered by their review, the use of salicylates (e.g. aspirins) for self-poisoning had declined, while that of paracetamol had increased (Proudfoot and Park, 1978).

Ghodse surveyed drug problems handled by sixty-two of London's sixty-six casualty units during one month in 1975. Altogether 1,641 parasuicides involving drug overdoses were recorded:

> 'Barbiturates were the commonest drug used by men and minor tranquillisers by women. However, when barbiturates are grouped with other non-barbiturate hypnotics, the most common drug used in self-poisoning was some kind of hypnotic or 'sleeper'. Minor tranquillisers were the second commonest group of drugs followed by aspirin/codeine compounds . . . About half of the men under the age of thirty-five took more than one drug, while for those between thirty-five and fifty-five there was an even greater incidence of polydrug overdose. Among the women there were more cases of single drug overdose than of polydrug overdose, although over the age of thirty years there was a greater tendency to take more than one drug . . . More than a quarter of the patients seen with a drug-related problem were thought to be dependent on drugs, either definitely or probably.' (Ghodse 1976)

As noted in the preceding chapter, barbiturate prescription has been drastically curtailed during the past decade. The steady replacement of barbiturates by the 'safe' benzodiazepines has been reflected by an equally steady decrease in both fatal and non-fatal overdoses involving such drugs. A review by Johns (1977) suggested that between 1959 and 1974 more than 27,000 people died of poisoning from self-administered barbiturates in England and Wales. Such deaths peaked in 1969 at 40 per million of the total population. Since then they have declined, although even during 1978 there were 790 deaths attributed to barbiturate poisoning in England and Wales. In addition, concern persists about the apparently disproportionately large number of those deaths attributed to Tuinal, which is also known to be a popular 'street' drug taken for kicks. In 1978 282 deaths were associated with this apparently very toxic drug. Paracetamol deaths are also a cause for concern. It has been widely noted that both parasuicides and suicides often involve overdoses of combinations of alcohol and other drugs. As noted in Chapter 2, such mixtures can have unexpectedly powerful and dangerous effects.

It is by no means certain precisely how many deaths are directly attributable to drug overdose of various types. For example, between 1982 and 1985 the annual number of deaths in the UK attributable to the misuse of glues and solvents has been estimated as rising from 60 to 114. It is likely that such estimates are understatements rather than true assessments of the real death toll due to either intentional or accidental drug poisoning.

Misuse of prescribed tranquillisers and sleeping pills

Most prescribing of tranquillisers and sleeping pills is fully justified and very valuable. Such preparations are now indispensable tools for coping with anxiety, depression and loneliness. The most conspicuous misuse of these freely available substances is in relation to overdoses. As noted above, even the relatively safe benzodiazepines can be taken for overdoses if sufficient quantities are accessible. There is no doubt that preparations such as Ativan, Librium and Valium are much less dangerous generally than barbiturates. Even so, the benzodiazepines do have a dependence-producing potential. During the early 1970s it was speculated that many thousands of people (mainly middle-aged women) were dependent upon prescribed barbiturates. Even today barbiturates continue to be dispensed in enormous quantities and it is probable that a minority of those receiving such drugs remain dependent upon them. A leading article in *The Lancet* in 1973 cogently drew attention to the disadvantages of the benzodiazepines.

'Experience dictates that whenever a new class of sedative drugs becomes available they are widely used until unwanted effects are belatedly discovered. This pattern, which is certainly not peculiar to psychopharmacology, was set with the bromides, barbiturates, and ineprobamate. But nothing has equalled the extent to which the benzodiazepines have been used . . . in the USA diazepam (Valium) prescriptions have been increasing by 7 million annually. At this rate the arrival of the millennium would coincide with the total tranquillisation of America. This is, of course, a general upward trend in all drug use, part of which is happily accounted for by more patients seeking or being able to obtain help. But the increase in consumption of benzodiazepines is both disproportionate to the rest of psychoactive drug use and absolute in that it does not reflect a switch from older or more dangerous drugs, the use of which has remained steady for several years . . . Anxiety certainly deserves to be treated; the idea that patients need to experience such suffering owes more to the puritan ethic than to psychoanalytical (or any other) theory. At the same time, extensive prescription of drugs for a condition that often improves spontaneously, or responds to reassurance or a simple placebo, may fairly often be called misuse . . . A self-fulfilling sequence is initiated, the more drugs are used, the more they seek to work, so the more they are prescribed.'

Even the benzodiazepines can produce dependence if prescribed in excessive amounts or for prolonged periods. Some patients appear to expect to use such drugs as long-term props. Some doctors allow them to do so and thereby, wittingly or unwittingly, collude in the creation of drug dependence. The numbers of those dependent upon prescribed sleeping pills and tranquillisers are unknown. Possibly the reduction in barbiturate prescribing has improved the situation. It may not have done, since the total quantities of psychoactive drug prescriptions continue to rise steadily. It is a very real dilemma how a balance is to be struck between meeting a genuine need for tranquillity and using drugs unnecessarily or even harmfully.

Roughly one million people in Britain take Valium. Many certainly manage to stop taking this drug without problems. Recent research indicates that a minority of users, possibly 2–5%, exhibit the symptoms of physical dependence on Valium, even after receiving only 'normal' doses. In some cases physical dependence becomes evident after taking Valium for as little as six weeks. Lader (1981) has suggested that 250,000 people in Britain are dependent upon tranquillisers or sleeping tablets. The corresponding number in the United States is estimated to be one million (Petursson and Lader 1981).

The following account of withdrawal from such drugs was published in *The Observer* (1980):

'One day I was in the supermarket and the lights were very bright. They seemed to flicker and I felt as though I was going to have a fit but instead I passed out. A doctor friend said that the lights were stimulating the bit of the brain that sometimes triggers a fit. Something must have made it extra sensitive. I couldn't believe what was happening to me. I'd got the shakes. I couldn't stop trembling. I had palpitations and perspired. Then there was the terrible muscle cramps. My neck and face were very tense and everything seemed an irritant.

I dragged myself through the day. It would be time to take a child to school or collect or something, and I'd just take half a tablet to calm me down so I could cope.

This was what happened when Jane, an articulate and lively woman in her mid-thirties tried to stop taking the tranquilliser Valium after about eighteen months on a normal dose of 30 mg a day . . . it took me months – yes months, with an s.

These were the physical symptoms of drug withdrawal. It was not all in the mind, not a psychological craving, not the anxiety coming back to me. Really I was addicted. It was a dreadful vicious circle. I had to keep on taking just one tablet to stave off the terrible feelings.' (Doyle 1980)

Tranquillisers, like alcohol, are depressants. In many ways it is socially acceptable for middle-aged women to use tranquillisers in much the same way that some men use alcohol. Tranquillisers do sometimes produce dependence and are certainly a cause of some road accidents, although to an unknown extent. The dangers of dependence upon these drugs have until recently been underestimated. Even the benzodiazepines can be at least as 'addictive' as heroin. It has been suggested in America that such dangers need to be described by an obligatory health warning similar to that on cigarette packets. Tranquillisers and sleeping pills are undoubtedly invaluable weapons against anxiety. Even so, their potential disadvantages are becoming all too apparent. One can only guess at the scale of dependence upon them and the psychological and social consequences of having millions of people partly or totally sedated by these preparations.

Postscript

In most countries, accidents are the most common cause of death amongst people aged thirty or under. The spread of the AIDS virus has already pushed accidents into second place in some American cities. Recent evidence (Robertson 1986) indicates that most intravenous drug users in Edinburgh and many of those in Dundee have been exposed to the AIDS virus. This ominous development could drastically change the risks of some forms of illegal drug use.

7 What Becomes of Drugtakers?

The widespread use of alcohol and tobacco has led to a greater public willingness to differentiate between their users than between illicit drugtakers. While it is conceded that a *minority* of drinkers and smokers do become 'hooked' or otherwise suffer from their drinking and smoking, illicit drugtaking has often been judged far more harshly. One popular view is that even casual experimentation involves a major risk of eventual drug dependence (the 'escalation' or 'stepping stone' theory). Another widely popularised belief is that opiate use involves an inevitable decline towards total degradation and premature death. Probably the only valid generalisation about drugtaking is that generalisations about it are invalid. The earlier chapters of this book have indicated that psychoactive drugs have very varied effects and are used for many reasons, and in many situations, by all manner of people. Few of those who use drugs correspond to the traditional stereotypes of either the 'alcoholic' or the 'junkie'. Even most of those who experience problems with drugs do not fit these over-simple and extreme images.

It is still widely believed that drug dependence is, if not incurable, virtually so. In addition it has often been emphasised that to 'recover' from drug dependence perpetual abstinence is essential. Due to the profusion of motivations, contexts and users it is not surprising that these beliefs are now shown to be erroneous. There is a large body of evidence indicating that an individual's pattern of drug use, or even the drug problems experienced, often change at different times. Indeed, some recent authorities suggest that both drug use and drug dependence often follow a natural course, albeit a highly variable one.

General patterns of use

It is worth repeating that while many reasons appear to explain why specific people use specific drugs at certain times, most drug use is attributable to social and cultural factors. The majority of recreational drug use (including that of alcohol, tobacco and the illicit drugs) is prompted by peer pressure. Most people use whatever drugs are in vogue among their friends and closest associates. It is also evident that because drugtaking is so heavily dependent upon the dictates of social acceptability (within one's own circle of acquaintances), it is constrained accordingly. Most people have workaday commitments, jobs and families. Drugtaking is generally restricted so that it does not interfere with primary obligations. An office worker appearing drunk on the job, or a student 'stoned' in lectures would rapidly be confronted with censure or mockery in consequence. Most drugtaking is a facet of leisure. It is part of 'time out' and usually an aid to relaxation. The rules of leisure are different from those of work. At a party one may quite acceptably get 'high' (often but not necessarily, with the aid of alcohol), flirt and engage in a wide variety of behaviour unthinkable during working time. Drugtaking is largely indulged in as a pleasure-producing activity. Individuals who, under the influence of drugs, become obnoxious or interfere with the enjoyment of others will usually be treated with disapproval or disdain by their associates. Such general rules of conduct apply as much to illicit drugtakers as to drinkers and smokers. Partly because of such social constraints and partly because most people have no wish to be perpetually under the influence of drugs, the majority of drugtakers enforce a strict division between drugtaking and other activities. Most drugtaking is sporadic, moderate and discreet. The overwhelming majority of alcohol consumption and illicit drugtaking occurs during leisure time. Cigarette smoking is different. Tobacco is the only drug that is widely used at work and in virtually all public places. People smoke on buses, in the street, at conferences, in factories and in offices. The social acceptability of such widespread smoking is declining, but still enables this 'portable addiction' to thrive. Whereas most forms of drug dependence are held in check by the social inappropriateness of frequent drug use, cigarette smoking still retains a unique level of social acceptance. This, combined with the high addiction producing potential of tobacco, has established tobacco dependence as the most widespread form of all drug dependence. Most alcohol, benzodiazepines, LSD or heroin users do not become drug dependent. Most tobacco smokers do.

There are many important common features between the long-term outcomes of using alcohol, tobacco, illicit drugs or prescribed drugs. There are also some significant differences. In order to clarify these, and before presenting general conclusions, each of these distinct forms of drug taking will be discussed separately.

Drinkers and problem drinkers

It has already been explained that most people drink in moderation and that the sensible consumption of alcohol appears to have definite benefits. Surveys show that most teenagers begin drinking regularly before they are eighteen and that people do their heaviest drinking while they are young and unmarried. It has also been noted in Chapter 6 that problem drinking, particularly public drunkenness, is largely but not exclusively, a young man's game. In contrast it is still true that the average age of those seeking professional help for alcohol problems is above forty. Young people seldom have had time to become physically dependent upon alcohol. The type of problems experienced by young drinkers are mainly associated with weekend drunkenness and are different from the longer-term type of difficulties which beset most middle-aged problem drinkers.

Most people who drink excessively or harmfully when they are young and single drastically reduce their levels of alcohol consumption when they are older or when they marry. Surveys have revealed that many people report having been heavy drinkers or even 'problem drinkers' when they were younger. While even young people may experience or inflict tragedies due to only a single drunken spree, it is reassuring to find abundant and clear evidence that most youthful excessive drinking is only temporary.

The traditional Alcoholics Anonymous (AA) view of 'alcoholism' is that it is incurable and can only be kept at bay by abstinence. As emphasised earlier in this book, 'alcoholism' is probably not a useful term. People may experience all manner of alcohol problems (or none) and even those diagnosed as 'alcoholics' by treatment agencies are a very varied group of people. Contrary to the established AA view, some people who have been identified as 'alcoholics' subsequently continue drinking, but at a moderate, controlled and harm-free level (Miller and Munoz 1976, Armor *et al.* 1978, Heather and Robertson 1986).

Innumerable studies have followed up the progress of identified problem drinkers. 'Success' rates vary enormously between different studies. In spite of this it is clear that a substantial percentage of problem drinkers given help by agencies of various types do resolve their problems, either by abstaining or by controlling their drinking. On average it seems that roughly one third of problem drinkers improve, one third deteriorate and one third remain relatively stable. Some studies report much better levels of 'success' than this, around 70–80%. The fact that a substantial percentage of problem drinkers do succeed in cutting their drinking either down or out is encouraging. This is particularly so since many doctors and nurses appear still to believe that problem drinkers cannot be helped and that attempting to do so is futile.

A particularly reassuring discovery is that the great majority of those in the community who experience alcohol problems manage to surmount their difficulties without recourse to professional help. These 'spontaneous remissions' have been the subject of considerable interest recently. Several British and American studies have concluded that many people with alcohol problems succeed in moderating their drinking for the following reasons:

1 Because their spouses, lovers, etc, put 'extreme pressure' on them to do so: 'If you don't stop getting drunk I'm going to leave you.'
2 Because a driving accident or other dramatic incident serves to convince them of the need to change.
3 Because of other important motivating pressures. Some people cut their drinking down when they fall in love, move to a new area, find new interests and new friends. Others do so because they have an important reason to ensure that their alcohol consumption is moderate. A professional driver, for example, cannot afford to lose his or her driving licence. A happily married person will not want drinking to damage his/her family life.

It is clear that informal social pressures often do succeed in persuading or forcing people to stop drinking excessively. Coercion seems much more constructive in relation to drinking problems than toleration, which may only perpetuate them.

The high mortality rate of problem drinkers is well known. As described earlier, some die of liver cirrhosis or in traffic accidents. Suicide is far more common among those with alcohol problems than among moderate drinkers. Evidence suggests that the likelihood that a problem drinker will 'do well' depends largely upon the personal characteristics of the individual. Those who have the greatest social and economic support appear to be better able than the socially bereft to overcome alcohol problems. The prognosis for people with friends, jobs, a home, money and loving support is better than for those who lack or who have already lost such things. Those with severe physical impairment (including possibly brain damage) or with clear-cut mental illnesses are less equipped to adapt their established patterns of harmful drinking than those without such handicaps.

It is evident that whatever advice is given to problem drinkers some will abstain, some will moderate their drinking and others will continue to drink in a damaging way. It must be emphasised that at present it is not possible to predict with certainty how an individual will respond, even though those least impaired by their drinking appear those most likely to resolve their problems. In particular it cannot safely be predicted which (minority) of those with alcohol problems are the ones who will manage to *control* their drinking. All that is apparent is that some people do succeed in doing this and will do so even if advised to abstain completely.

Cigarette smokers

Two important features distinguish cigarette smoking from all other types of drugtaking. First, the majority of those who smoke, even those who have only recently started to do so, appear to want to give it up eventually. Secondly, very few smokers can be classified as only intermittent or occasional. Most are regular smokers and most are psychologically and physically dependent upon tobacco.

The major health risks associated with smoking are all too well documented and have been summarised in Chapters 2 and 6. As described in Chapter 5 there has been a decline in smoking in the United Kingdom during recent years. Many people have given up the practice and have done so without professional help. In fact, professional help to give up smoking has only become available very recently and remains extremely limited. In 1979 survey data showed that 51% of male current smokers were smoking at least twenty cigarettes daily. The corresponding percentage of female smokers was 35%. Set against this very high level of heavy smoking was the fact that 27% of males and 14% of females aged sixteen and above reported that they had smoked in the past, but did not do so at present. Very clearly some people do manage to stop smoking, even if only temporarily. Some of these appear to abstain successfully, while others would be forced to agree with Mark Twain that giving up smoking is easy. They have done it dozens of times.

The success of treating cigarette-dependent people has been reviewed by Raw. This review concluded that, in general, under 15% of cigarette smokers are able to stop permanently before they are sixty years old:

'A person who has become a regular smoker is very unlikely to be able to stop, and the fairly low long-term success rates of treatment programmes testify to this fact also.' (Raw 1978)

Raw's review of current evidence revealed that the average level of success in giving up smoking achieved by people helped to do so in twenty studies was roughly 20%.

Illicit drugtakers

Most of those who use illicit drugs do so only in a very limited way and for a relatively short period. Surveys have shown that illicit drugtaking, like heavy drinking, is mainly a pastime of young, unmarried people, especially those living away from their parental homes and mixing mainly with other young people.

As described in Chapter 5, most illicit drugtaking occurs in the form of communal cannabis smoking at social gatherings such as weekend parties. The evidence from field research suggests that many young people who use illicit drugs may experiment with several substances and be quite regular users of some (especially cannabis) for two or three years. It is clear that while many of those smoking cannabis also experiment with other drugs such as LSD and amphetamines, only a minority use opiates and the great majority would not countenance the injection of heroin or any other drug. It is true that many opiate dependants report that their drugtaking careers started with cannabis (and alcohol, tobacco and gripe water). Similarly, people identified as problem drinkers report that they started drinking socially. Just as social drinking obviously does not lead most people to experience serious alcohol problems, so cannabis smoking does not, in itself, involve a high level of risk of eventual opiate dependence. Millions of people have used cannabis without either using or being attracted to opiates or drug injection.

It has long been popularly assumed that the opiates are highly addictive, so that even one or two experiences of such drugs will lead to dependence. In fact it is now clear that some people use opiates only sporadically or intermittently without becoming dependent upon them. Such users have been colloquially referred to in drug scene jargon as 'chippers'. In addition, it is now demonstrated that people may use heroin and allied drugs regularly and for some time without necessarily experiencing any major or problematic withdrawal symptoms. This has been widely reported and the most dramatic example of the cessation of opiate use was provided by the returning American service personnel who had served in Vietnam. It was known that opiate use was extremely widespread among American troops involved in the Vietnam War and this prompted concern that these people would remain dependent on these drugs after their return to America. In addition it was assumed that treatment facilities would be required to assist these opiate dependants through the rigours of withdrawal, or to wean them away from heroin to 'preferable' alternatives such as methadone.

The experience of the Vietnam opiate users was examined by Robins (1978) in what is certainly one of the most interesting and impressive pieces of recent drug research. Robins found that service in Vietnam provided a unique setting to foster drug use. The proportion of troops in her study who reported having used narcotics was 48%. Follow-up research, including blood tests to detect the presence of opiates, showed that 95% of the Vietnam opiate users stopped using such drugs when they returned to America. Most of these men stopped opiate use immediately they returned and few reported experiencing much difficulty or discomfort in relinquishing the habit. Robins' study showed that while in Vietnam the pressures and situation gave huge opportunity and provided great pressure to use opiates. For this reason those who did use these drugs were not distinctive from non-users in relation to their family backgrounds, criminal records and previous alcohol and other drug problems. Such traits only distinguished the minority who continued to use drugs upon their return to the USA. Sadly a large number of Vietnam veterans have subsequently developed problems related to alcohol and drugs. Many have committed suicide or have become mentally ill. It has been estimated that of the 2,600,000 American service personnel who served in Vietnam, 800,000 (32%) are suffering from 'post-traumatic stress disorders' (Brende and Parson 1985).

The experience of these Vietnam opiate users is exceptional. No studies of clinic populations of opiate users have produced levels of remission as high as

95%. Even so, it is clear that many people use opiates in a very casual way without necessarily becoming dependent. In addition it is also clear that a substantial proportion of heroin dependants in clinics eventually cease or reduce their opiate use. A ten year follow-up study of 128 heroin users attending London drug dependence clinics revealed 35% had stopped using opiates. In addition it was discovered that such abstinence had not apparently been replaced by dependence on other drugs. Set against this, 12% had died and 48% were still using opiates, although in some cases this use appeared to be only sporadic (Stimson and Oppenheimer 1982).

There is an extensive literature on the prognosis of institutionalised opiate users. This indicates that, on average, such individuals have a mortality rate of one to two percent per year (Thorley 1981, Raistrick and Davidson 1985, Bucknall and Robertson 1986). Some British agencies, such as the City Roads Crisis Intervention Centre in London, note higher levels of client deaths (Jamison, Glanz and Macgregor 1984). A review of Ghodse *et al.* (1985) concluded that between 1967 and 1981, 1,499 'notified addicts' had died. This mortality exceeds that of the general population of comparable age and sex by 16 times. AIDS could completely alter this picture.

Users of prescribed tranquillisers and sleeping pills

Very little indeed is known about what becomes of users of prescribed preparations such as Librium and Valium. As explained in the previous chapter some users take overdoses and some become dependent. Such outcomes are not surprising among people who are depressed, lonely or unhappy. It is clear that great care is needed to limit the misuse of such drugs. Even so, one can only speculate about the extent of problems related to these very widely used psychoactive substances.

Some general conclusions about what happens to drugtakers

As the preceding account indicates, drug dependence or the experience of drug problems need not be permanent. Many people who at some stage in their lives experience such difficulties, resolve them later on and usually do so without professional help. As described in Chapters 5 and 6 most drugtaking does not involve either becoming dependent or experiencing serious problems. In addition, most drugtakers adapt their styles of drug use to meet the demands of a 'normal life'. With the exception of cigarette smoking (in relation to which heavy or dependent use is normal) most drugtaking does not in itself appear to be a problem, except of course in relation to the illegal status of certain practices.

There is a considerable body of evidence that most of those who experience problems with alcohol or illicit drugs eventually 'mature out' of their difficulties spontaneously. In addition, such remissions mainly happen either because a new circle of relationships and interests makes drugtaking less important or because strong social pressures encourage an active reduction in drugtaking. Many people use even the most 'dangerous' substances such as glues, LSD and opiates without apparent harm. It is also evident that many people who become dependent upon drugs subsequently manage to abstain or to reduce their drug use sometimes without experiencing the major discomforts previously thought to be inevitable accompaniments of withdrawal.

Does 'treatment' help?

Probably it does. Possibly it makes little difference to the natural course of a person's drugtaking career. There is no evidence suggesting that one specific type of treatment achieves notably better results than alternatives. All manner of approaches are used to assist people with drug problems (psychoanalysis, behaviour therapy, family therapy, Synanon, 'born-again' Christianity, Alcoholics Anonymous, abstinence, controlled drinking, Scientology, Divine Light, Buddhism, acupuncture, transcendental meditation, 'concept houses' and a variety of religious conversions).

Many treatment approaches have never been evaluated. Even so, those working in such agencies are generally optimistic that they do help a substantial percentage of their clients to overcome their problems. In view of the diversity of people with so many varied drug problems, it is not surprising that such a wide range of types of help exists and that each of these appears to be helpful to some people. Very often people manage to overcome drug problems by finding new friends and new interests. This may happen spontaneously. Such a process may also be aided by the 'artificial' provision of a new reference group, social support and new values. Alcoholics Anonymous and many religious cults help some people to abandon drug use largely because they give a satisfying alternative to it.

In addition they provide another focus for people's affiliative needs. They offer new friends, values and prestige, all of which may be vital inducements to giving up or cutting down drug use. Evaluations of treatment approaches for alcohol, tobacco and illicit drug problems show that there is little to choose between the overall effectiveness of the wide variety of helping approaches available. In addition it appears that out-patient treatment is as effective as in-patient care. Voluntary or 'amateur' counsellors appear to have as much to offer as trained professionals. From all this it should be accepted that all approaches probably have something to offer to some people with drug problems. Conversely, no single approach seems suitable for all such people. The majority of those who contact any agency will probably not respond well to whatever it offers them. Many will go elsewhere and some will drop out of whatever programme is offered them. Even so, evidence shows that a substantial proportion, although probably a minority, of those given help are successful in either ceasing or reducing their drug use. The majority will survive, even if they do not achieve marked reductions in drug use.

It is possible that those who do manage to overcome drug dependence or drug problems do so largely because of the type of people they are and the amount of social support available to assist them. Some cynics have suggested that treatment, counselling, etc. for drug problems probably does little good, since those people who are going to 'make it' will do so anyway. This may be so, in some cases at least. Very often people moderate their drinking, opiate use, etc. because they form new relationships or enter new social settings. Most student cannabis smokers, for example, certainly reduce or abandon cannabis use when they qualify and enter professional groups in which only alcohol and to a (much) lesser extent, tobacco, are approved drugs. Many helping agencies cannot provide new lifestyles. Some, of course, such as AA are able to do this. Others appear to be useful motivating forces to facilitate change. Even though the *precise* value of various types of help is not clear, it is evident that many of those who have drug problems will be able to change their behaviour in the desired direction. It is therefore manifestly worthwhile and rewarding to continue to assist such changes.

Drugtaking (except for tobacco smoking) does not in itself imply a major risk of eventual dependence. There is no inevitable *escalation* from one form of drugtaking to more harmful types. At the same time, drug dependence or drug problems are often only temporary and the majority of those who do succeed in overcoming drug problems do so spontaneously and without the help of treatment agencies.

8 What Can Be Done?

The scale of drug problems is enormous and some drug problems are increasing relentlessly. It is of very great importance, therefore, to consider what, if anything, can be done to prevent such problems arising. Several alternative strategies have been suggested and this chapter reviews some of the merits and limitations of possible courses of action.

Education: A mixed blessing

Most discussions of drug problems culminate in a plea for 'more' or 'better' health education to prevent people from developing drug problems. Obviously it would be a vast improvement if people could, at an early age, be 'taught' about the properties and potential dangers of drugs and become thereafter non-smoking, moderate drinkers. In fact very little public money is spent on health education in Britain. The Health Education Council and the Scottish Health Education Group have to operate on a tiny fraction of the money that is available, for example, to advertise alcohol, tobacco or prescribed drugs. Even at this crude level, the 'competition' appears to be a very unequal one.

Due to severe financial constraints, health education activities have been limited. During recent years some television, newspaper and poster campaigns have been mounted and a number of educational aids such as films, audiotapes, booklets and leaflets have been produced. Examples of recent health education posters on excessive drinking and cigarette smoking are depicted in Figures 8.1, 8.2 and 8.3.

Many health education activities have been directed at specific target groups such as schoolchildren. Others have been aimed more generally at the population in certain areas (such as Tyneside or Scotland). A major problem besetting health education is that of identifying objectives in relation to drugtaking. Most people now assume that the aims of 'official' campaigns should be (a) to discourage cigarette smoking and illicit drug use, and (b) to foster moderate or restrained alcohol use. These aims are prompted by the

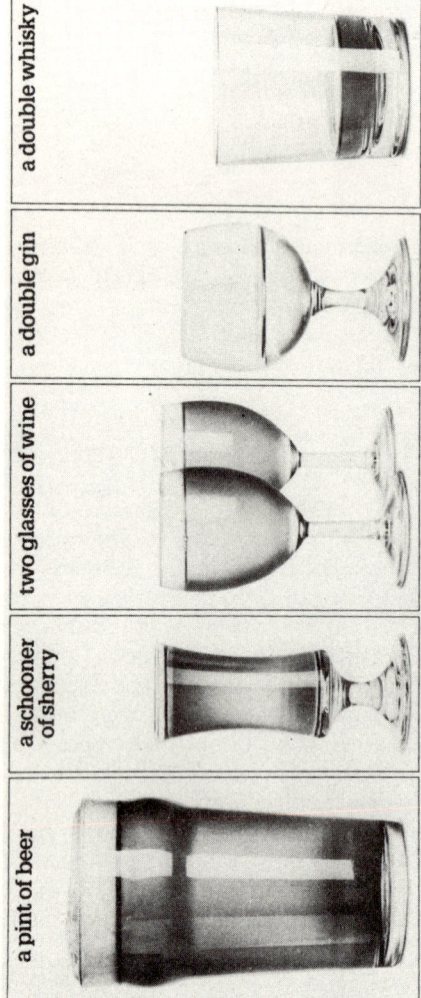

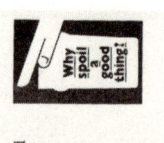

Fig. 8.1 *It's all the same to your liver*

Fig. 8.2 *No wonder smokers cough*

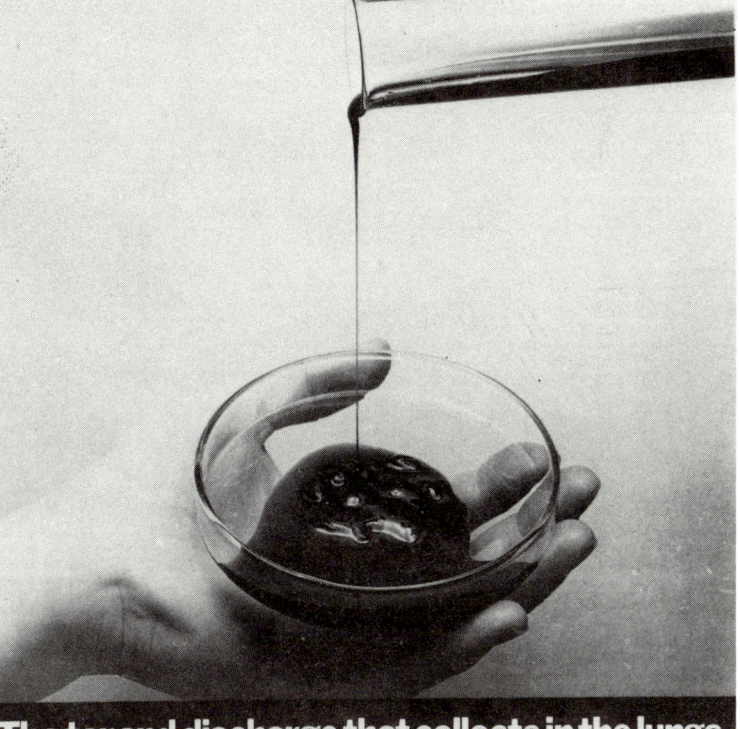

Fig. 8.3 *Smoking gets right up other people's noses*

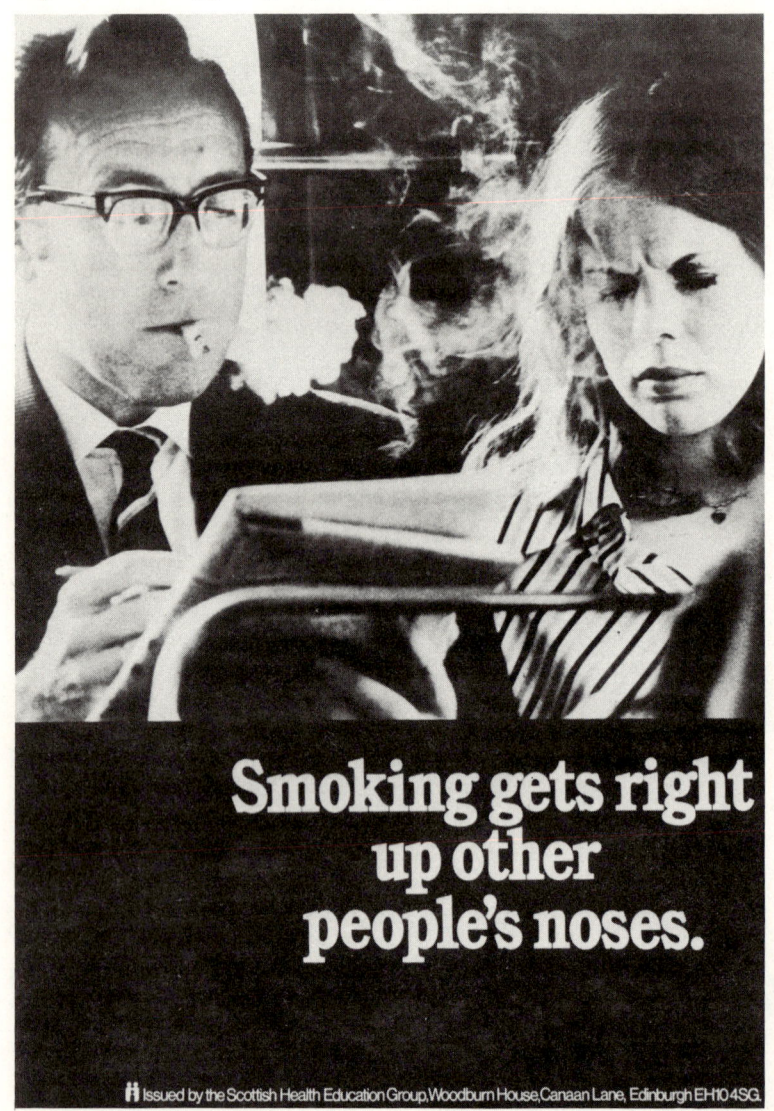

facts that smoking kills people and illicit drugtaking is either illegal or lacks widespread social support. In addition it is generally conceded that most alcohol use is moderate and beneficial and that even if it were not it *has* considerable social support. Most people drink and few campaigns attempt to promote abstinence from alcohol. In fact these objectives are all controversial. There is not a monolithic consensus about the aims of drug education. Some people believe that campaigns should attempt to discourage even moderate drinking. Conversely, others believe that illicit drugtaking is not in itself harmful and that it is more realistic to urge not abstinence but responsible or sensible use and to minimise the harm associated with drug use. Even the objective of discouraging people from smoking is hotly contested by some people and of course by the tobacco products manufacturers.

Voluntary codes of advertising practice have been introduced which restrict the types of advertising appeal used to popularise alcoholic drinks or tobacco products. These codes have certainly led to a moderation of such advertising. It has been suggested that there should be a total ban on advertising tobacco and alcohol. This might make the task of health educationalists easier. Even so, it must be recognised that in countries such as those in Eastern Europe where such advertising is already banned, drug problems seem to have continued to increase. It is doubtful that further curbs on advertising would produce dramatic results, and evidence on the effects of alcohol and tobacco advertising is sparse and equivocal.

It does appear that the highly publicised reports on smoking by the Royal College of Physicians led at least to a short-term fall in tobacco use by the general population. Smoking has been declining recently and it is reasonable to attribute at least part of this decline to heightened public awareness of the dangers of cigarettes. Other educational 'successes' have related to the curtailment of prescribing amphetamines and then barbiturates. Apart from these encouraging examples, there is little cheer around. Dorn (1981) concluded that 'no known method of drug education can be said to reduce drug use'. In addition important reviews of alcohol and drug education by Kalb (1979), Kinder, Pape and Walfish (1980), Schaps *et al.* (1981) and Bandy and President (1983) have reached generally depressing conclusions. These suggest that such educational activities mainly appear to have been ineffective or, in some cases, may have been *counterproductive*. Equally worrying is evidence that the more young people know about illegal drugs, the *safer* they regard such substances as being (Glaser and Snow 1969, Swisher 1971).

Pickens (1983) reviewing information-based drug education evaluations, concludes that such activity:

'will have most impact if it coincides with the period of development during which young people both begin to make significant use of legal drugs and start to have significant degrees of contact with illegal drugs. Before this stage drug education will be irrelevant – after it will be ineffective'.

A review of English language studies of the effects of tobacco education has also produced rather sombre conclusions. Thomson (1978) concluded that:

> 'Most methods used with youth have shown little success. Studies of other methods have shown contradictory results. The two methods showing most promise are individual counselling and smoking withdrawal clinics'.

Some studies have drawn promising conclusions, although it is emphasised that these are greatly outnumbered by those which have not done so. For example, McAlister *et al.* (1980) concluded that junior high school students in California who were trained to resist pressure to use alcohol, tobacco and illegal drugs were less likely to use these substances, or to use them often, as other students who had not experienced such training. The Royal College of Physicians (1983) concluded that although non-smoking campaigns appear to produce only transient effects, they do serve to draw public attention to health risks and to reinforce negative images of smoking. Aaro *et al.* (1983) and Gillies and Willcox (1984) have reported encouraging results from educational initiatives related to smoking. The latter study indicated that nine to eleven year old children exposed to tobacco education were less likely to begin to smoke than comparable children who had not received such education. More recently Gillies, Pearson and Elwood (1986) have noted that amongst 15–16 year olds in the Trent Regional Health Authority area, those who recalled having had tobacco education were slightly more likely to smoke than were those who had not had such education. The researchers cautioned that this difference does not necessarily imply that tobacco education led to smoking.

> 'The finding is likely to have resulted from problems of recall and discrepant reporting'.

Sometimes 'health education' related to drugs, alcohol and tobacco is a mixture of education (the provision of factual information) and propaganda (an organised scheme to propagate a doctrine or practice). During 1985 and 1986 the British Government initiated an expensive 'anti-drug campaign' which included television advertisements. In England and Wales the campaign involved the negative portrayal of the possible effects of heroin use. This is exemplified by Figure 8.4. The Scottish counterpart of this campaign, mounted by the Scottish Health Education Group, avoided such a negative approach and is illustrated by Figure 8.5 The concept of a national anti-drug campaign has been widely criticised on the grounds that such costly exercises seldom appear to be effective and that they risk increasing

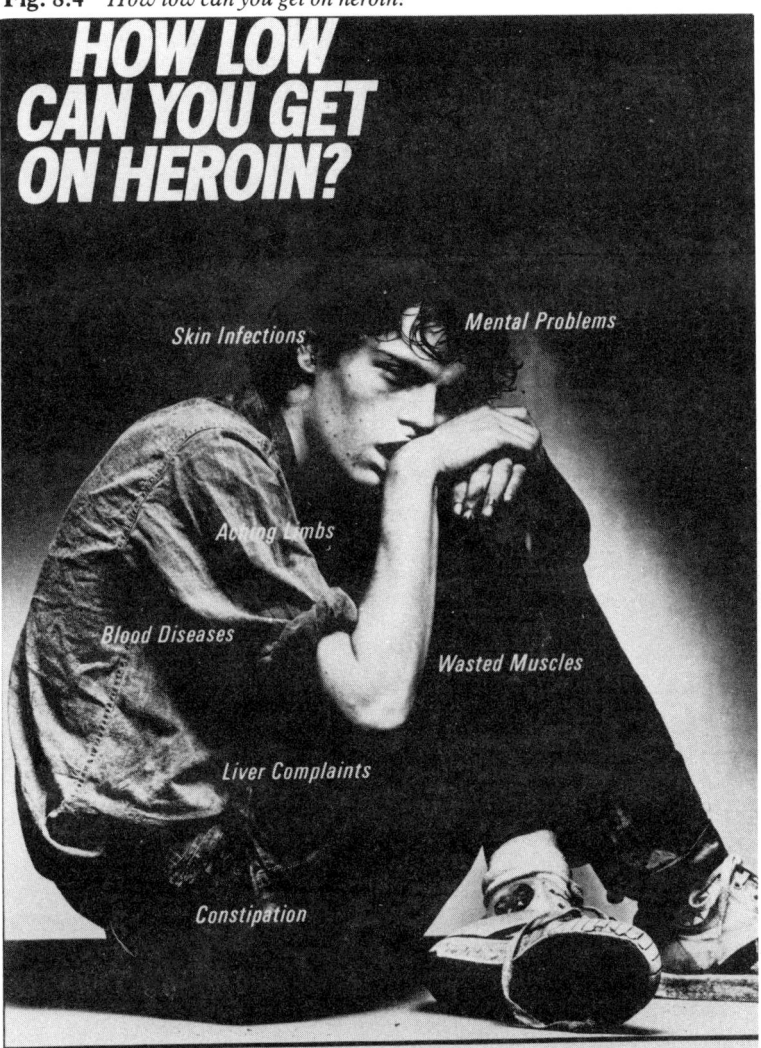

Fig. 8.4 *How low can you get on heroin?*

Fig. 8.5 *Choose life, not drugs*

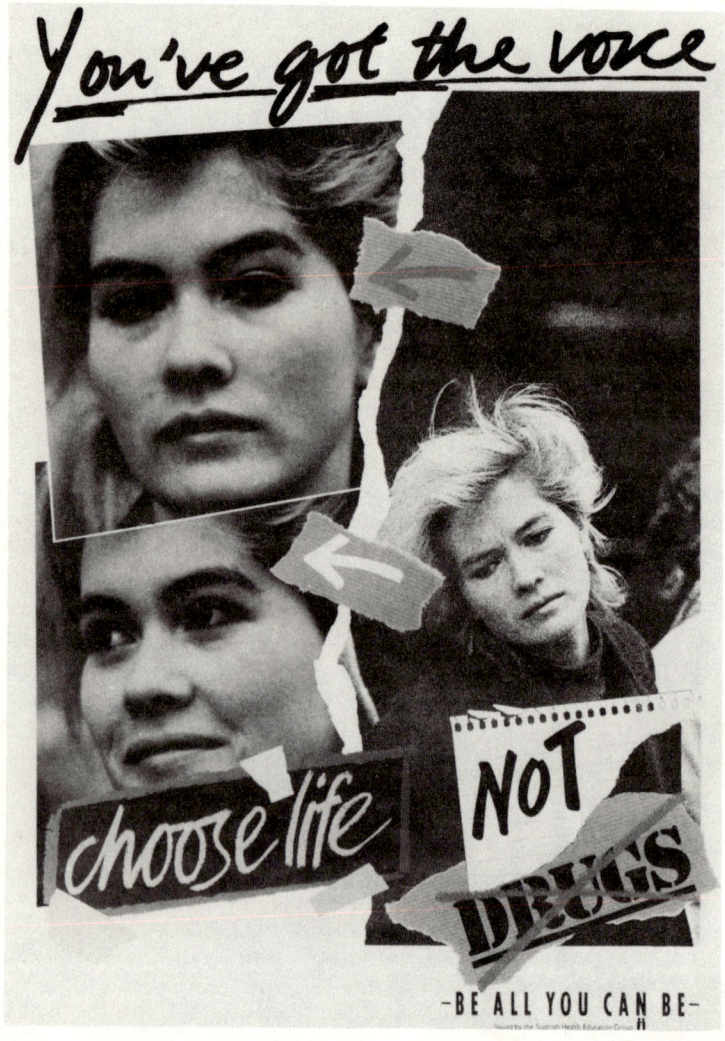

interest in drug use with possibly adverse consequences (Advisory Council on the Misuse of Drugs 1984, leading article British Medical Journal 1985). Marsh (1986) has concluded that the anti drug campaign in England and Wales was 'evaluated' in such an inadequate way that it is not possible to assess its effects, if any.

Health education is potentially important. Even so, in relation to alcohol, tobacco and prescribed drugs, it must be regarded as purely experimental and should be approached cautiously and with due regard to the evidence that it may be ineffective or harmful. Nobody would seriously suggest that mass inoculation should be attempted with a dubious vaccine. A similar restraint is needed in relation to health education. Future initiatives should be conducted with a far greater degree of awareness of the limitations and potential damages of such endeavours. At present a surprising number of practitioners appear to be unaware of the disappointing past experience in this field.

It may be unrealistic to expect that health education, at least in the short-term, will lead to significant behaviour changes in the general population. Such changes may be unattainable or may take a very long time to occur. Humans are not rational, Vulcan-like beings. In consequence, it does not follow that improved levels of knowledge alter attitudes or that changed attitudes necessarily influence behaviour. Education cannot be conducted in a vacuum. It is widely assumed or hoped that drug education will discourage people from using drugs. It would be possible to improve general levels of factual knowledge about drugs, but this may have the opposite effect from that of prevention. Educational campaigns have, however, been good at encouraging people with alcohol or other drug problems to seek help. The effectiveness of health education can really only be judged in the long term. The absence of evidence of short-term changes on drug use in its varied forms may not imply that health education does not work. Even so, it must be acknowledged that there is at present very little evidence that educating people about drugs leads to more sensible drugtaking or to fewer drug problems.

Very often 'health education' has been limited to showing a film to schoolchildren. Frequently such education has been confined either to a one-off lecture by a visiting 'expert' such as a policeman or doctor. Alternatively, schools in particular have thrust the responsibility of providing drug education on to a hapless teacher who is already fully committed with academic work and who does not always know much about drugs or who is hardly an example in relation to his/her own drinking and smoking. It clearly is as silly for teachers who smoke to warn young people of the dangers of this practice as it is for parents who smoke to do so. Many schools now accept that health education is a proper part of the curriculum, and some have begun to include such material at the secondary level. This is admirable and sensible. At present it must be concluded that there is not a properly formulated drug educational policy in Britain. It is not generally agreed which are the right target groups (schoolchildren, parents, workers?) or which methods are the most efficient. There is evidence that showing 'horror films' about the extreme ill effects of drug misuse does not produce the desired results. Educational appeals must above all be designed so that specific target groups can identify with the material presented. Twelve-year-old schoolchildren do not identify with gangrenous heroin injectors or middle-aged tramps imbibing meths. In addition drug education must be accurate. Many teenagers no longer believe that smoking cannabis inevitably leads to drug dependence. The experiences of their friends inform them differently. For these reasons health education should adopt a factual, non-moralising approach that provides people with useful and relevant information designed to meet the needs of specific target groups. It is also currently believed that drug education in schools should be raised not as a separate issue in isolation from other topics, but should be part of the broader curriculum. This sounds fine, but in practice often means that little or no drug education is provided.

A major limitation of drug education is that there is little evidence that many people get into trouble with drugs through lack of knowledge. Doctors and nurses working in lung cancer wards presumably know that smoking kills people, yet some continue to smoke. As reviewed in Chapter 2, people use drugs for many complex reasons. The main single *cause* of drugtaking appears to be social pressure to do so. People generally derive their ideas about drugs from those with whom they identify and those with whom they associate. Lectures by visiting 'experts' or thirty-second televised commercials may well be like water off a duck's back in relation to the influence of such informal social cues. In relation to illicit drugtaking, there is evidence that initial use is often preceded by conversion to the idea that drugtaking is safe. Most drugtakers appear to be at least averagely intelligent and many know a great deal about the effects of specific drugs.

Sometimes education can be directed through unorthodox channels. In the past information about the dangers of some types of drugtaking (such as amphetamine and barbiturate injection or the use of 'Angel Dust') has been made effectively available through the 'underground press'. Such publications, while in general being sympathetic to drugtaking, have often highlighted warnings if evidence suggested certain practices to be dangerous. Their warnings appear to have been especially authoritative because it was known that they were not inspired by a general dislike of drug use.

Illicit drugtaking is often at least partly inspired by rebelliousness and a wish to flout 'established values'. Health education is closely identified with conventional wisdom, and may, in relation to illicit drug use, be ineffective for this reason. In addition, health education can hardly be expected to compensate for some of the factors reviewed in Chapter 2 which sometimes foster drugtaking.

Health education is an important activity and has an important symbolic value as an arm of public policy. It is valuable in highlighting important issues and priority target groups such as school children and the medical profession. The existence of drug education promotes awareness of the importance of drug problems as a matter for public concern and public policy. In addition drug education certainly increases the likelihood that public policies will be constructive and humane.

It took decades for changing fashion to achieve a reduction in smoking.

Possibly progress in relation to other forms of drugtaking will take at least as long to become apparent.

Much health education activity related to drugs has been concerned with imparting information about the potential dangers of certain drugs. This in reality is probably not the main requirement. It might be more useful in relation to illicit drugtaking to clarify the role of drugs as a symbol of youthful rebellion or as a means of coping with personal problems. It would also be logical to develop discussion of what alternative ways are available to express rebellion or to contend with problems.

Evidence suggests that some sub-groups of children are more at risk of developing drug problems than others. Within school, truants and educational failures might be usefully picked as high priority groups who might be especially vulnerable to the seductions of their local drug scene. Educational activities should be more influenced than they often have been by the many pressures promoting drugtaking and in particular of those pressures that sometimes cause excessive or harmful drug use or drug dependence. Serious consideration needs to be given to providing education to minimise the risks of certain forms of drug use. The advent of AIDS as a possible consequence of intravenous drug use makes this a crucial public health issue.

Restricting drug availability

In general the extent of drug problems relates closely to the level of drug use. Some social groups suffer much higher rates of drug problems than others and some drugs are much more dangerous than others. Even so, the more drugtakers there are the greater is the chance that some people will use drugs harmfully or will become dependent upon them. As stated in Chapter 1, different societies have varied attitudes to drugs. A substance that is revered in one country is reviled elsewhere. There is little rhyme or reason in the choice by any society of which drugs are safe. The use of drugs that are socially disapproved of, such as cannabis or opiates in Britain, is penalised and it is widely accepted that it is a justified and crucial social policy to restrict the availability of such substances. In consequence a considerable amount of activity by the police, Customs and Excise, the courts and penal institutions is devoted to enforcing the drug control laws.

The massive health damage caused by smoking has led to an increase in pressure for advertising of tobacco products to be limited, and the (minor) restriction of smoking in some public places and modes of transport. On health grounds it has been generally accepted that people should ideally not smoke at all. Alcohol consumption is different since drinking is not in itself harmful (quite the reverse), only excessive drinking provides a cause for concern. There is indisputably a relationship between the average or general level of alcohol consumption and rates of alcohol problems. This has not been defined mathematically, and is subject to all manner of social, economic, psychological and other influences. In consequence control of the overall level of alcohol consumption has recently been urged as a logical means of attempting to stabilise or reduce the rates of alcohol problems (e.g. Royal College of Psychiatrists 1979, 1986). This strategy is essentially a *political* problem. Roughly 90% of British voters drink alcohol, even if only occasionally. Stabilising or cutting the general level of alcohol consumption would require a substantial increase in the price of alcoholic drinks. There is little doubt that such a step would have the desired effect upon alcohol problems, although to what extent is uncertain. Such action, though certainly sensible from a public health point of view, would certainly face huge political opposition. Even relatively trivial increases in the price of alcohol and tobacco have been unpopular in the past.

Rigorous price manipulation or other measures aimed at limiting the general extent of drug use are only feasible if they have sufficient public support. In addition there are many reasons apart from the total level of consumption why any drug is sometimes misused. It is certain that some types of drug misuse are more attributable to traditional attitudes and social conditions than simply to the total quantities of any substances that are used.

Control measures all have disadvantages. Under the existing drug laws thousands of young people are involved in court proceedings every year due to largely innocuous cannabis smoking. One might well conclude that the present law in this respect causes far more distress and damage than cannabis itself appears to do. Even so, the law reflects popular sentiment, which is why some drugs are deemed acceptable and others are not. Historically, attempts at drug control, ranging from Prohibition in the United States to opiate controls throughout the world have all produced some undesirable consequences. Whenever a substance is proscribed a black market springs up to meet whatever demand for this substance exists. Sometimes a vicious and criminal situation develops and illicit supplies may be of dubious purity. The main disadvantage of 'extreme' control measures is that they drive drugtakers underground and make drug use firstly a crime and secondly furtive and at odds with society. Ultimately decisions on the price, legal status and availability of drugs are made in the ballot box, or by opinion polls.

Other strategies

The misuse of drugs could also be approached by attempting to control not the general level of drugtaking but by severely penalising dangerous or anti-social behaviour such as drunken driving or publicly obnoxious behaviour under the influence of drugs. Other countries (such as Norway) are far more thoroughgoing than the UK in relation to controls on drunken driving. In addition there is plenty of scope for extending existing laws on public drunkenness or of more fully enforcing existing laws.

None of the approaches discussed in this chapter is likely to be a magic solution. All doubtless have merit and all are to some extent compatible. A country may justifiably use all of these approaches if deemed appropriate. Clearly the ideal and least painful strategy would be the educational approach. This would be far more palatable than using either price controls or strict legal sanctions. Even so, health education appears unlikely to make more than a partial incursion into the total level of drug problems, since so many of these appear due to profound social and psychological factors beyond the control of educationalists.

9 Conclusions

It must be emphasised that this book is not just about drug problems. It is also about drug use. The massive popularity of psychoactive drugs to allay depression or to enhance relaxation is a measure of their value to humanity. This fact is easily overlooked when confronted with the all too tragic evidence of social, psychological and physical harm caused by the misuse of drugs. It is much easier to measure and describe the disadvantages and harm associated with drugs than to assess or to explain their advantages.

Most people choose to use drugs at least sometimes. Drug use is a firmly established and important adjunct to many social activities. In addition tranquillisers and sedatives are indispensable weapons against mental illness. It is probable that the demands for such preparations will continue to rise as medicine is increasingly expected to help people overcome unhappiness or to provide a buffer against social isolation. Many drug problems cannot be quantified. Nobody is in a position to do more than speculate upon the numbers of people who use drugs excessively or harmfully. The 'cost' of drug misuse is certainly huge but unknown. The number of accidents caused by middle-aged women 'stoned' on benzodiazepines is uncertain. Even the numbers of deaths due to cigarette smoking can only be gauged in very rough terms.

The huge popularity of drugs and the extensive problems associated with them present a difficult choice for any society. People must pay for their pleasures. If it is agreed that people have a right to cheap mass-produced drugs it must also be ensured that any consequent problems will be responded to effectively. An Exchequer which annually accrues over £5,700,000,000 from alcohol and £5,000,000,000 from tobacco revenue can reasonably be expected to provide adequate funds for drug education and research and for the provision and evaluation of services to help those with drug problems. At present much of the burden of providing such services is placed upon agencies with pitifully small resources. It is admirable that unpaid volunteers and self-help organizations should be active in helping those with drug problems. There will always be a need for such selfless voluntary activity but the increased scale of drug problems should be matched by a corresponding increase in services to cope with such problems. At present many agencies such as counselling services, detoxification centres, hostels and clinics are facing closure due to lack of public financial support.

It is arguable that a considerable proportion of existing public expenditure on drug-related projects and services is wasted. Most of the agencies receiving public funds have never been evaluated or been made to justify their existence. Many health education activities have similarly been accepted uncritically. Increased public spending in this field would be a logical response to drug problems especially if such spending was to be aimed at preventing the emergence of future drug problems. The complete range of public activities in this field needs, as a matter of priority, to be critically evaluated. Which techniques work best? Which are the cheapest and serve to help the greatest number in need?

Even if public spending is to be limited there is a need to examine the effectiveness of whatever activities are financed. Health education, as emphasised above, cannot be judged solely by short-term criteria. Attitudes to alcohol, tobacco, illicit drugs and prescribed drugs have taken decades, if not centuries, to develop. It may take as long to change or to 'improve' these attitudes. There is plenty of scope for further research to identify which people are especially likely to experience drug problems and the situations or other factors that foster such problems. If society demands psychoactive drugs it must be prepared to meet the costs of the levels of drugtaking that are deemed appropriate. Drugs and humanity appear to be inseparable.

Appendix I

Some Useful Addresses – United Kingdom and Eire

Compiled by Mrs Ray Stuart, Alcohol Research Group, Department of Psychiatry, University of Edinburgh.

Sources of information

Action on Alcohol Abuse (AAA)
  Livingstone House
  11 Carteret Street
  London SW1H 9DL
  01 222 3454

Alcohol Concern
  305 Gray's Inn Road
  London WC1X 8QF
  01 833 3471

Association for the Prevention of Addiction (APA)
  54/56 New Oxford Street
  London WC1A 1ES
  01 580 0580
  (General information)

Institute for the Study of Drug Dependence
  1/4 Hatton Place
  Hatton Gardens
  London EC1N 8ND
  01 430 1991–2–3
  (Information about research literature)

Standing Conference on Drug Abuse (SCODA)
  1/4 Hatton Place
  Hatton Gardens
  London EC1N 8ND
  01 430 2341–2
  (Information on help or treatment available nationally)

APPENDIX I

Standing Conference on Drug Abuse
266 Clyde Street
Glasgow G1
041 221 1175

Release
347a Upper Street
London N1 0PD
01 603 8654
(For information and legal help)

Teachers' Advisory Council on Alcohol and Drug Education (TACADE)
3rd Floor
Furness House
Trafford Road
Salford M5 2XJ
061 848 0351

Health Education Council (for England and Wales)
78 New Oxford Street,
London WC1 1AH
01 631 0930
(General information)

Scottish Health Education Group
Health Education Centre
Woodburn House
Canaan Lane
Edinburgh EH10 4SG
031 447 8044
(General information)

Health Education Service
16 College Street
Belfast 1
0232 241771

Health Education Bureau (Eire)
34 Upper Mount Street
Dublin 2
0001 762393
(General information)

Action on Smoking and Health (ASH)
5/11 Mortimer Street
London W1N 7RH
01 637 9843–6
(Smoking and health)

Scottish Committee (ASH)
6 Castle Street
Edinburgh EH2 3AJ
031 225 4725
(Smoking and health)

Scottish Council for Voluntary Organisations
18/19 Claremont Street
Edinburgh EH7 4QD
031 556 3882
(Produces a directory of residential facilities in Scotland)

South Wales Association for the Prevention of Addiction Ltd.
111 Cowbridge Road East
Cardiff CF1 9AG
0222 26113
(General information)

The Terrence Higgins Trust
BM/AIDS
London WC1N 3XX
01 833 2971
Open from 7–10 pm weekdays,
3–10 pm weekends.
(Advice on AIDS)

Drug treatment agencies

The majority of psychiatric hospitals provide help for individuals with drug problems. Local information can usually be obtained from family doctors or from social work departments. Most towns have at least one agency that can help with alcohol or other drug problems. The following is by no means a complete list, and further information can be obtained either from some of the above addresses or from some of those below.

A directory of drug services for Scotland is available from the Scottish Health Education Group. A similar register, related to England and Wales, is available from the Standing Conference on Drug Abuse.

The following addresses are those either of drug treatment centres, or of hospitals where doctors are licensed to prescribe heroin and allied drugs.

ENGLAND

Avon
Bristol Royal Infirmary
 Marlborough Street
 Bristol BS2 8HW
 0272 22041

APPENDIX I

Bedfordshire
Luton and Dunstable Hospital
  Lewsey Road
  Luton LU4 0DZ
  0582 573211

Buckinghamshire
St John's Hospital
  Stone
  Aylesbury HP17 8PP
  0296 748383

Cambridgeshire
Addenbrookes Hospital
  Psychiatric Outpatients
    Department
  2 Benet Place
  Lensfield Road
  Cambridge CB2 1EL
  0223 66461

Peterborough District Hospital
  Thorpe Road
  Peterborough PE3 6DA
  0733 67451

Cheshire
Countess of Chester Hospital
  Mersey Regional DDC
  Chester CH2 1BQ
  0244 390333

Thomas Percival Unit
  Winwick Hospital
  Winwick
  Warrington WA2 8RR
  0925 55221

Halton Drug Dependency Unit
  The Rear
  39–41 Victoria Road
  Widnes WA8 7RP
  051 423 5247

Warrington Drug Dependency
Clinic
  9 Wilson Patten Street
  Warrington WA1 1LZ
  0925 415176

Cleveland
St Lukes Hospital
  Psychiatric Department
  Marton Road
  Middlesbrough TS4 3AF
  0642 813166

Cornwall
Royal Cornwall Hospital (City)
  Ward 9
  Infirmary Hill
  Truro TR1 2HZ
  0872 74242

St Lawrences Hospital
  Bodmin PL31 2QT
  0208 3281

Cumbria
Garlands Hospital
  Garlands
  Carlisle CA1 3SX
  0228 31081

Devon
Exminster Hospital
  Exminster EX6 88B
  0392 71337

District Drug Problem Team
  Belmont Court
  124 Newton Road
  Torquay TQ2 7AD
  0803 615741

Dorset
St Ann's Hospital
  Drug Abuse and Addiction Clinic
  Haven Road
  Carford Cliffs
  Poole BH13 7LN
  0202 708881

Essex
Rochford Hospital
  Daly's Road
  Rochford SS4 1RB
  0702 546393

Gloucestershire
Cheltenham General Hospital
  Psychiatric Unit
  Sandford Road
  Cheltenham GL53 7AN
  0242 580344

Hampshire
Knowle Hospital
  Fareham PO17 5NA
  0329 832271

Moorhaven Hospital
  Psychiatric Service
  Bittaford
  Ivybridge PL21 0EX
  0752 892411

Nuffield Clinic
  Psychiatric Day Centre
  Seventrees
  Lipson Road
  Plymouth PL4 8NQ
  0752 660281

Runwell Hospital
  The Chase
  Wickford S11 7QE
  03744 5555

Coney Hill Hospital
  Cheltenham Ward/Gloucester Ward
  Coney Hill
  Gloucester GL4 7QJ
  0452 617033

Royal South Hampshire Hospital DDC
  Department of Psychiatry
  Fanshawe
  Southampton SO9 4PE
  0703 34288

APPENDIX I

St James' Hospital
 High Clair DDU
 Milton
 Portsmouth PO4 8LF
 0705 822331

Hertfordshire
Hill End Hospital
 Hill End Lane
 St Albans AL4 0RB
 0727 55555

Kent
Bethlem Royal Hospital
 Drug Dependency Unit
 Monks Orchard Road
 Beckenham BR3 3XB
 01 777 6611

Bexley Hospital
 Ashdown Ward
 Old Bexley Lane
 Bexley DA5 2BW
 0322 526282

Leicestershire
Towers Hospital
 Humberstone
 Gypsy Lane
 Leicester LE5 0TD
 0533 767184

Greater London
Charing Cross Hospital
 Drug Dependency Unit
 57 Aspenlea Road
 London W6
 01 385 8834/5

Hackney Hospital
 Drug Dependency Unit
 Homerton High Street
 London E9 6BE
 01 986 6816

Basingstoke District Hospital
 Park Prewett
 Basingstoke RG24 9LZ
 0256 473202

Queen Elizabeth II Hospital
 Department of Psychiatry
 Howlands
 Welwyn Garden City AL7 4HQ
 07073 28111

Kent and Canterbury Hospital
 Ethelbert Road
 Canterbury CT1 3NG
 0227 66877

Ealing Hospital
 St Bernard's Wing
 Regional Alcoholism and
 Drug Dependency Unit
 Uxbridge Road
 Southall UB1 3QG
 01 574 2444

The London Hospital (St Clement's)
 Drug Addiction Unit
 2a Bow Road
 London E3
 01 377 7000

The Maudsley Hospital
  Drug Dependency Unit
  Denmark Hill
  London SE5 8AZ
  01 703 6333

St George's Hospital
  Drug Dependency Clinic
  Blackshaw Road
  London SW17 0QT
  01 672 1255

St Mary's Hospital
  Drug Dependency Clinic
  Praed Street
  London W2
  01 723 8829

Tooting Bec Hospital
  Drug Dependency Unit
  Tooting Bec Road
  London SW17 8BL
  01 672 9933

West Middlesex Hospital
  Drug Dependency Unit
  Twickenham Road
  Isleworth TW7 6AF
  01 560 2121

Great Chapel Street Medical Centre
  13 Great Chapel Street
  London W1V 7AL
  01 437 9360

Greater Manchester
Prestwich Hospital DDU
  Bury New Road
  Prestwich
  Manchester M25 7BL
  061 773 2236

Queen Mary's Hospital
  Drug Treatment Centre
  Roehampton Lane
  London SW15 5PN
  01 789 6611

St Bernards Hospital
  Drug Dependency Unit
  Uxbridge Road
  Southall UB1 3QG
  01 574 2444

St Giles Hospital
  Drug Dependency Clinic
  St Giles Road
  Camberwell
  London SE5
  01 703 0898

St Thomas' Hospital
  Drug Dependency Clinic
  Lambeth Palace Road
  London SE1
  01 633 0720

University College Hospital
  Drug Dependency Clinic
  122 Hampstead Road
  London NW1 2LT
  01 387 9300

Westminster Hospital DDC
  c/o St Stephen's Hospital
  Fulham Road
  London SW10
  01 352 8161

APPENDIX I

Merseyside
Hope Street Drug Dependence Unit
  30 Hope Street
  Liverpool L1 9BX
  051 709 0516

St Helens Hospital
  Psychiatric Dept.
  Marshals Cross Road
  St Helens WA9 3EA
  0744 26633

Southport Drug Dependency Clinic
  46 Houghton Street
  Southport PR9 0PQ
  0704 33133

Royal Liverpool Hospital
  Drug Dependency Unit
  Liverpool L7 8XT
  051 709 0141

St Catherine's Hospital
  Church Road
  Birkenhead L42 0LQ
  051 652 2281

Midlands
All Saints Hospital
  Lodge Road
  Birmingham B18 5SD
  021 523 5151

Norfolk
The Buer Centre (DDC)
  West Norwich Hospital
  Bowthorpe Road
  Norwich NR2 3UD
  0603 628377

Northamptonshire
St Crispin Hospital
  Duston
  Northampton NN5 6UN
  0604 52323

Nottinghamshire
Mapperley Hospital
  Addiction Unit
  Porchester Road
  Nottingham NG3 6AA
  0602 608144

Oxfordshire
Ley Clinic
  Littlemore Hospital
  Oxford OX4 4XW
  0865 778911

Shropshire
Royal Shrewsbury Hospital
  Shelton
  Bicton Heath
  Shrewsbury SY3 8XF
  0743 52244

Somerset
Mendip Hospital
  Bath Road
  Wells BA5 3DJ
  0749 72211

Yeovil District Hospital
  Higher Kingston
  Yeovil BA21 4AT
  09357 5122

Staffordshire
St George's Hospital Drug Clinic
  Milford Ward
  Personality Disorder Unit
  St George's Hospital
  Stafford ST1 3AG
  0785 57888 ext. 243

Surrey
Brookwood Hospital
  Knap Hill
  Woking GU21 2RQ
  04867 4545

Rees House Day Hospital
  Drug Dependency Clinic
  2/4 Morland Road
  Croydon CR0 6NA
  01 654 8100

Sussex
Herbert Hone Clinic
  Brighton Drug Dependency Unit
  11 Buckingham Road
  Brighton BN1 3RA
  0273 29604

Crawley Hospital
  West Green Drive
  Crawley RH11 7DH
  0293 27866

St Christopher's Day Hospital
  Hurst Road
  Horsham RH12 2EP
  0403 54367

APPENDIX I

Tyne and Wear
Cherry Knowle Hospital
 CADET
 Wellfield Clinic
 Ryhope
 Sunderland SR2 0LY
 091 5210541

North East Council on Addictions
 1 Mosley Street
 Newcastle on Tyne NE1 1YE
 0632 320797

West Midlands
'Aquarius'
 The White House
 111 New Street
 Birmingham B24 EU
 021 632 4722
 (Also centres in Dudley, Telford,
 Wolverhampton and
 Northampton).

Worcestershire
Worcester Royal Infirmary
 Community Drug Service
 Newtown Branch
 Newtown Road
 Worcester WR5 1JG
 0905 353507 or 353266

Yorkshire
Bootham Park Hospital
 63 Bootham Park
 York YO3 7BY
 0904 54664

St Mary's Hospital DDC
 Dean Road
 Scarborough YO12 7SN
 0723 376111

Royal Hallamshire Hospital
 Glossop Road
 Sheffield S10 2JF
 0742 26484

Parkwood House
 Alcohol and Drug Addiction Unit
 St Nicholas Hospital
 Gosforth
 Newcastle upon Tyne NE3 3XT
 0632 850151

Clifton Hospital
 Shipton Road
 York YO3 6RD
 0904 36661

Doncaster Royal Infirmary
 Psychiatric Unit
 Armthorpe Road
 Doncaster DN2 5LT
 0302 666666

Leeds Addiction Unit
 40 Clarenden Road
 Leeds LS2 9PJ
 0532 456617

Waddiloves Forensic Psychiatric
Unit
  44 Queen's Road
  Bradford BD8 7BT
  0274 497121

Northern General Hospital
  Sheffield S5 7AO
  0742 434343

WALES

Clwyd
North Wales Hospital
  Gwynant Ward
  Denbigh LL16 5S9
  074 571 2871

Gwent
St Cadoc's Hospital
  Caerleon NP6 1XQ
  0633 421121

Powys
Mid-Wales Hospital
  The Radnor Unit
  Talgarth
  Brecon LD3 0DS
  0874 711671

South Glamorgan
University Hospital of Wales
  Heath Park
  Cardiff CF4 4XW
  0222 755944

Whitchurch Hospital
  Whitchurch
  Cardiff CF4 7XB
  0222 62191

NORTHERN IRELAND

Antrim
Shaftesbury Square Hospital
  116–18 Great Victoria Street
  Belfast BT2 7BG
  0232 229808

Armagh
St Luke's Hospital
  Loughall Road
  Armagh BT61 7NQ
  0861 522381

APPENDIX I

Down
Downshire Hospital
 Ardglass Road
 Downpatrick BT30 6RA
 0396 3311

EIRE

Drug Advisory and Treatment Centre
 Jervis Street Hospital
 Dublin 1
 0001 748782

SCOTLAND

Ayrshire
Ailsa Hospital
 Dalmellington Road
 Ayr KA6 6AB
 0292 265136

Borders
Dingleton Hospital
 Melrose DD6 9HN
 089 682 2727

Central
Bellsdyke Hospital
 Larbert FK5 4SF
 0324 556131

Dumfries and Galloway
Crighton Royal Hospital
 Glencairn Ward
 Dumfries BG1 4TG
 0387 55301

Grampian
Kingseat Hospital
 Newmachar
 Aberdeenshire AB5 0NH
 065 17 2253

Royal Cornhill Hospital
 26 Cornhill Road
 Aberdeen AB9 2ZF
 0224 632411

Highland
Dunain House Addiction Unit
  Craig Dunain Hospital
  Inverness IV3 6JU
  0463 234101

Lothian
Royal Edinburgh Hospital
  Morningside Place
  Edinburgh EH10 5HF
  031 447 2011

Strathclyde
Duke Street Hospital
  253 Duke Street
  Glasgow G31 1HY
  041 554 6267

Leverndale Hospital
  510 Crookston Road
  Glasgow G51
  041 882 6255

Southern General Hospital
  1345 Govan Road
  Glasgow G51 4TF
  041 445 2466

Gartnaval Royal Hospital
  Ward 1a
  1053 Great Western Road
  Glasgow G12 0XH
  041 334 6241

Monklands District General Hospital
  Monkscourt Avenue
  Airdrie ML6 0JS
  023 64 69344

Woodilee Hospital
  Kirkintilloch
  Glasgow G66 3UG
  041 776 2451

Tayside
Wishart Drug Problems Centre
  61 King Street
  Dundee DD1 2GY
  0382 25083

Agencies helping with alcohol problems

There is a national network of National Health Service alcohol problems treatment agencies and of local councils on 'alcoholism'. These, together with Alcoholics Anonymous, Al-Anon and Al-Ateen groups, cover most of the country. Details of local facilities can be obtained from the following addresses.

APPENDIX I

ENGLAND

Alcohol Concern
305 Gray's Inn Road
London WC1X 8QF
01 833 3471

Alcoholics Anonymous
UK General Services Office
PO Box 514
11 Redcliffe Gardens
London SW10
01 352 9779
(Information about local AA groups)

Al-Anon Family Groups UK
61 Dover Street
London SE1 4YF
01 403 0888
(Information about Al-Anon groups for the families of problem drinkers)
Al-Ateen, which caters for adolescent children of problem drinkers, can also be contacted at 01 403 0888)

Medical Council on Alcoholism
1 St Andrews Place
London NW1 4LB
01 487 4445
(Education for doctors and nurses)

SCOTLAND

Scottish Council on Alcohol
147 Blythswood Street
Glasgow G2 4EN
041 333 9677
(For details of treatment agencies including local councils on alcoholism)

NORTHERN IRELAND

The Northern Ireland Council on Alcoholism
40 Elmwood Avenue
Belfast BT9 6AZ
0232 664434
(For details of treatment agencies)

EIRE

The Irish National Council on Alcoholism
 19–20 Fleet Street
 Dublin 2
 0001 774091
 (For details of treatment agencies)

Appendix II

Some recommended reading

CURRAN, V. and GOLOMBOK, S. (1985) *Bottling It Up*. London: Faber and Faber.
FREEMANTLE, B. (1985) *The Fix*. London: Corgi.
GOSSOP, M. (1982) *Living with Drugs*. London: Temple Smith.
HEATHER, N. and ROBERTSON, I. (1986) *Problem Drinking*. Harmondsworth: Penguin.
KREITMAN, N. (ed.) (1977) *Parasuicide*. Chichester: Wiley.
MORGAN, H. G. (1979) *Death Wishes? The Understanding and Management of Deliberate Self-Harm*. Chichester: Wiley.
PLANT, M. A. (ed.) (1982) *Drinking and Problem Drinking*. London: Junction/Fourth Estate.
PLANT, M. A., PECK, D. F. and SAMUEL, E. (1985) *Alcohol, Drugs and School-Leavers*. London: Tavistock.
PLANT, M. L. (1985) *Women, Drinking and Pregnancy*. London: Tavistock.
ROYAL COLLEGE OF PHYSICIANS. (1983) *Health or Smoking?* London: Pitman.
ROYAL COLLEGE OF PSYCHIATRISTS. (1986) *Alcohol: Our Favourite Drug*. London: Tavistock.
STIMSON, G. V. and OPPENHEIMER, E. (1982) *Heroin Addiction*. London: Tavistock.
TAYLOR, P. (1984) *Smoke Ring: The Politics of Tobacco*. London: Bodley Head.

Bibliography

The following bibliography lists the main references found to be useful while writing and revising this book. Most are not cited directly in the text. Readers requiring a select reading list of useful and easily obtainable references are referred to the list above.

AARO, L. E., BRULAND, E., HAUKNES, A. and LOCHSEN, P. M. (1983) 'Smoking among Norwegian school children 1975–1980, III. The effect of anti-smoking campaigns.' *Scandinavian Journal of Psychology*, 24, pp. 1–7.
ADLER, M. W. (1986) 'AIDS and intravenous drug users'. *British Journal of Addiction*, 81, pp. 307–310 (editorial).
ADLER, P. (1985) *Wheeling and Dealing: An Ethnography of an Upper-level Drug Dealing and Smuggling Community*. New York: Columbia University Press.
ADVERTISING ASSOCIATION. (1986) *Statistics Yearbook 1985*. London: Advertising Association.

ADVISORY COUNCIL ON THE MISUSE OF DRUGS. (1982) *Treatment and Rehabilitation*. London: Department of Health and Social Security.

ADVISORY COUNCIL ON THE MISUSE OF DRUGS. (1984) *Prevention*. London: Home Office.

ALTMAN, D. (1986) *AIDS and the New Puritanism*. London: Pluto.

ARMOR, D. J., POLICH, J. M. and STAMBULL, H. B. (1978) *Alcoholism and Treatment*. Chichester: Wiley.

ARMYR, G., ELMER, A. and HERZ, V. (1982) *Alcohol in the World of the 80's*. Stockholm: Sober Forlags A.G.

BAKALOR, J. B. and GRINSPOON, L. (1984) *Drug Control in a Free Society*. Cambridge: Cambridge University Press.

BANDY, P. and PRESIDENT, P. A. (1983) 'Recent literature on drug abuse and prevention and mass media: focusing on youth, parents, women and the elderly'. *Journal of Drug Education*, 13, pp. 255–271.

BANKS, A. and WALLER, T. A. N. (1983) *Drug Addiction and Polydrug Abuse*. London: Institute for the Study of Drug Dependence.

BEBBINGTON, P. E., (1976) 'The efficacy of Alcoholics Anonymous; the elusiveness of hard data'. *British Journal of Psychiatry*, 128, pp. 572–580.

BELL, C. G. and BATTJES, R. (eds) (1985) *Prevention Research: Deterring Drug Abuse Among Children and Adolescents*. Rockville, Maryland: NIDA Monograph 63, National Institute on Drug Abuse.

BENJAMIN, C. (1979) 'Persistent psychiatric symptoms after eating psilocybin'. *British Medical Journal*, 1, (6174), pp. 1319–1320.

BERNARD, G. (1983) 'An economic analysis of the illicit drug market'. *International Journal of the Addictions*, 18, pp. 681–700.

BERRIDGE, V. (1979) 'Opium in the fens of nineteenth century England'. *Journal of the History of Medicine*, July, pp. 293–313.

BERRIDGE, V. and EDWARDS, G. (1981) *Opium and the People*. London: Allen Lane.

BETHUNE, H. (1985) *Off the Hook*. London: Methuen.

BINNIE, H. L. and MURDOCH, G. (1969) 'The attitudes to drugs and drug takers of students of the university and colleges of higher education in an English Midland city'. University of Leicester, *Vaughan Papers*, 14, pp. 1–29.

BLACK, D. (1986) *The Plague Years: A Chronicle of AIDS, the Epidemic of Our Time*. London: Picador.

BLACKWELL, J. (1983) 'Drifting, controlling and overcoming: opiate users who avoid becoming chronically dependent'. *Journal of Drug Issues*, 12, pp. 219–235.

BLANE, H. T. and CHAFETZ, M. E. (eds) (1979) *Youth, Alcohol and Social Policy*. New York: Plenum.

BLUM, R. H., GARFIELD, E. F., JOHNSTONE, J. L. and MAGISTAD, J. (1978) 'Drug education: further results and recommendations'. *Journal of Drug Issues*, 8, pp. 379–426.

BOSTOCK, Y. and DAVIES, J. K. (1979) 'Recent changes in the prevalence of cigarette smoking in Scotland'. *Health Bulletin*, 37, pp. 260–267.

BREEZE, E. (1985a) *Differences in Drinking Patterns Between Selected Regions*. London: HMSO.

BREEZE, E. (1985b) *Women and Drinking*. London: HMSO.

BRENDE, J. O. and PARSON, E. R. (1985) *Vietnam Veterans: The Road to Recovery*. New York: Plenum.

BREWERS' SOCIETY. (1986) *U.K. Statistical Handbook*. London: Brewers' Society.

BRITISH MEDICAL ASSOCIATION. (1986) *Young People and Alcohol*. London: British Medical Association.

BRUNN, K., PAN, L. and REXED, I. (1979) *The Gentleman's Club: International Control of Drugs and Alcohol*. Chicago: Chicago University Press.
BUCKNALL, A. B. V. and ROBERTSON, J. R. (1985) 'Heroin misuse and family medicine'. *Family Practice*, pp. 244–251.
BUCKNALL, A. B. V. and ROBERTSON, J. R. (1986) 'Deaths of heroin users in a general practice'. *Journal of the Royal College of General Practitioners*, 36, pp. 120–122.
BUCKNALL, A. B. V., ROBERTSON, J. R. and STRACHAN, J. G. (1986) 'Use of psychiatric drug treatment services by heroin users from general practice'. *British Medical Journal*, 292, pp. 997–999.
BUCKNALL, P. and GHODSE, H. (1986) *Misuse of Drugs*. London: Waterloo.
BURR, A. (1984) 'The illicit non-pharmaceutical heroin market and drug scene in Kensington Market'. *British Journal of Addiction*, 79, pp. 337–344.
CAHALAN, D. (1970) *Problem Drinkers: A National Survey*. San Francisco: Jossey-Bass.
CAMBERWELL COUNCIL ON ALCOHOLISM. (eds) (1980) *Women and Alcohol*. London: Tavistock.
CANADIAN GOVERNMENT COMMISSION OF INQUIRY. (1971) *The Non-medical Use of Drugs*. Harmondsworth: Penguin.
CAPLIN, S. and WOODWARD, S. (1986) *Drugwatch: Just Say No*. London: Corgi.
CARTER, M. (1976) 'Will the legal liberty cap cause Home Office hallucinations?' *New Scientist*, 71, pp. 599.
CARTWRIGHT, A. K. J., SHAW, S. J. and SPRATLEY, T. A. (1978) 'The relationships between per capita consumption, drinking patterns and alcohol-related problems in a population sample 1965–1974. Part 1: Increased consumption and changes in drinking patterns.' *British Journal of Addiction*, 73, pp. 237–46.
CENTRAL POLICY REVIEW STAFF. (1979) *Alcohol Policies in the United Kingdom* (The 'Think Tank Report'). Stockholm: Sociologiska Institutionen, Stockholms Universitat (Printed in 1982).
CHAMBERS G. and TOMBS, J. (eds) (1984) *The British Crime Survey Scotland, A Scottish Office Research Study*. Edinburgh: HMSO.
CHARLTON, A. (1984) 'Children's coughs related to parental smoking'. *British Medical Journal*, 288, pp. 1647–1649.
CLARK, J. P. and TIFFT, L. (1966) 'Polygraph and interview validations of self-reported deviant behaviour'. *American Sociological Review*, 31, pp. 516–523.
CLAYSON, C. (1972) *Report of the Departmental Committee on Scottish Licensing Law*. Edinburgh: HMSO.
COCKETT, R. (1971) *Drug Abuse and Personality in Young Offenders*. London: Butterworths.
COHEN, S. (1972) *Folk Devils and Moral Panics*. London: Granada.
COLEMAN, V. (1977) *The Medicine Men*. London: Arrow.
COLLINS, J. J. JNR. (ed.) (1982) *Drinking and Crime*. London: Tavistock.
CONNOLLY, G. N., WINN. D. M., HECHT, S. S. *et al*. (1986) 'The reemergence of smokeless tobacco'. *New England Journal of Medicine*, 314, pp. 1020–1027.
CORDER, B. W., SMITH, R. A. and SWISHER, J. D. (1985) *Drug Abuse Prevention*. Dubuque, Iowa: Wm. C. Brown.
COURTWRIGHT, D. T. (1982) *Dark Paradise*. Cambridge, Mass.: Harvard University Press.
COX, T. C., JACOBS, M. R., LEBLANC, A. E. and MARSHMAN, J. A. (1983) *Drugs and Drug Abuse: A Reference Text*. Toronto: Addiction Research Foundation.
CRAWFORD, A., PLANT, M. A. KREITMAN, N. and LATCHAM, R. (1984) 'Regional variations in alcohol-related morbidity in Britain: A myth uncovered? II. Population survey'. *British Medical Journal*, 289, pp. 1343–1349.

CRAWFORD, A. and PLANT, M. A. (1986) 'Regional variations in alcohol dependence rates: A conundrum'. *Quarterly Journal of Social Affairs*, 2, pp. 139–144.

CURRAN, V. and GOLOMBOK, S. (1985) *Bottling It Up*. London: Faber and Faber.

DANIELS, V. G. (1986) *AIDS: Questions and Answers*. Cambridge: Cambridge Medical Books.

DAVIES, D. L. (1962) 'Normal drinking in recovered alcoholics'. *Quarterly Journal of Studies on Alcohol*, 23, pp. 94–104.

DAVIES, P. T. and WALSH, D. (1983) *Alcohol Problems and Alcohol Control Policies in Europe*. London: Croom Helm.

DE ALARCON, R. and RATHOD, N. H. (1968) 'Prevalence and early detection of heroin abuse'. *British Medical Journal*, 2, pp. 549–553.

DE LINT, J. (1975) 'Current trends in the prevalence of excessive alcohol use and alcohol-related health damage'. *British Journal of Addiction*, 70, pp. 3–14.

DEPARTMENT OF HEALTH AND SOCIAL SECURITY. (1985) *Health and Personal Social Services Statistics for England and Wales 1985 Edition*. London: HMSO.

DEWHURST, K. (1980) 'Psilocybin intoxication'. *British Journal of Addiction*, 137, pp. 303–304.

DIGHT, S. (1976) *Scottish Drinking Habits*. London: HMSO.

DOBBS, J. and MARSH, A. (1983) *Smoking Among Secondary School Children*. London: Office of Population Censuses and Surveys, HMSO.

DORN, N. (1981) 'Social analysis of drugs in health education and the media', In: Edwards, G. and Busch, C. (eds) *Drug Problems in Britain*. London: Academic Press.

DORN, N. (1983) *Alcohol, Youth and the State*. London: Croom Helm.

DORN, N. and SOUTH, N. (1985) *Helping Drug Users*. London: Gower.

DOYAL, L. and EPSTEIN, S. S. (1983) *Cancer in Britain*. London: Pluto.

DOYLE, C. (1980) 'The dangers of tranquillity'. *Observer Living*, Sunday, 24th Feb., p. 45.

DRUMMOND, L. M. (1986) 'Cannabis psychosis: A case report'. *British Journal of Addiction*, 81, pp. 139–140.

DUFFY, J. and PLANT, M. A. (1986) 'Scotland's liquor licensing changes: an assessment'. *British Medical Journal*, 292, pp. 86–39.

DYER, J. (1980) 'Self poisoning: the magnitude of the problem'. *Personal Communication*.

EASTMAN, C. (1984) *Drink and Drinking Problems*. London: Longman.

EDWARDS, G. (1971) *Unreason in an Age of Reason*. Edwin Stevens Lectures for the Laity, London, Royal Society of Medicine.

EDWARDS, G. (1982) *The Treatment of Drinking Problems*. London: Grant McIntyre.

EDWARDS, G. (1984) 'Drinking in longitudinal perspective: career and natural history'. *British Journal of Addiction*, 79, pp. 179–184.

EDWARDS, G., ARIF, A. and JAFFE, J. (eds) (1983) *Drug Use and Misuse: Cultural Perspectives*. Beckenham: Croom Helm/World Health Organization.

EDWARDS, G., CHANDLER, J. and HENSMAN, C. (1972) 'Drinking in a London suburb'. *Quarterly Journal of Studies on Alcohol*, 6, pp. 69–93.

EINSTEIN, S. (1975) *Beyond Drugs*. London: Pergamon.

ERROLL OF HALE. (1971) *Report of the Departmental Committee on Liquor Licensing*. London: HMSO.

EVANS, C. (1985) 'Preliminary findings: Survey on drug use by young people in Tower Hamlets youth clubs and youth centres'. London Borough of Tower Hamlets, Directorate of Social Services, Information Pack V (unpublished).

FAGIN, L. and LITTLE, M. (1984) *The Forsaken Families*. Harmondsworth: Penguin.

FAZEY, C. (1977) *The Aetiology of Psychoactive Substance Use*. Paris: Unesco.
FIELD, T. (1985) *Escaping The Dragon*. London: Unwin.
FISH, F., WELLS, B. W. P., BINDEMAN, G., BUNNEY, J. E. and JORDAN, M. M. (1974) 'Prevalence of drug misuse amongst young people in Glasgow, 1970–1972'. *British Journal of Addiction*, 69, pp. 231–236.
FREEMANTLE, B. (1985) *The Fix*. London: Corgi.
FURST, P. T. (1976) *Hallucinogens and Culture*. San Francisco: Chandler and Sharp.
GABE, J. and WILLIAMS, P. (eds) (1986) *Tranquillisers: Social, Psychological and Cultural Perspectives*. London: Tavistock.
GHODSE, H. (1976) 'Drug problems dealt with by 62 London casualty departments'. *British Journal of Preventive and Social Medicine*, 30, 4, pp. 251–6.
GHODSE, H., SHEEHAY, M., TAYLOR, C. and EDWARDS, G. (1985) 'Deaths of drug addicts in the United Kingdom 1962–1981'. *British Medical Journal*, 290, pp. 429–428.
GILLIES, P., PEARSON, J. C. G. and ELWOOD, J. M. (1986) 'Survey of smoking in 15–16 year olds'. Nottingham: Department of Community Health, University of Nottingham.
GILLIES, P. and WILLCOX, B. (1984) 'Reducing the risk of smoking amongst the young'. *Public Health*, 98, pp. 49–54.
GLANZ, A. and TAYLOR, C. (1986) 'Findings of a national survey of the role of general practitioners in the treatment of opiate misuse: extent of contact with opiate misusers'. *British Medical Journal*, 293, pp. 427–430.
GLASER, D. and SNOW, M. (1969) *Public Knowledge and Attitudes to Drug Use*. New York: Addiction Control Commission.
GLYNN, T. J. (ed.) (1983) *Drug Abuse Prevention Research*. US Department of Health and Human Services, Research Issues No. 33, Rockville, National Institute on Drug Abuse.
GODFREY, C., HARDMAN, G. and POWELL, M. (1986) 'Alcohol, tobacco and taxation'. *British Journal of Addiction*, 81, pp. 143–150.
GOODE, E. (1970) *The Marijuana Smokers*. New York: Basic Books.
GOODE, E. (1972) *Drugs in American Society*. New York: Alfred A. Knopf.
GOODE, E. (1973) *The Drug Phenomenon: Social Aspects of Drug Taking*. New York: Bobbs-Merrill Co. Inc.
GOODWIN, D. (1976) *Is Alcoholism Hereditary?* New York: Oxford University Press.
GOSSOP, M. (1982) *Living with Drugs*. London: Temple Smith.
GRANT, M. (1984) *Same Again*. Harmondsworth: Pelican.
GRANT, M. (ed.) (1985) *Alcohol Policies*. Copenhagen: World Health Organization.
GRANT, M. and GWINNER, P. D. V. (eds) (1979) *Alcoholism in Perspective*. London: Croom Helm.
GRANT, M., PLANT, M. A. and WILLIAMS, A. (eds) (1983) *Economics and Alcohol*. London: Croom Helm.
GREENBLATT, M. and SCHUCKIT, M. (eds) (1976) *Alcoholism Problems in Women and Children*. New York: Grune and Stratton.
GUSFIELD, J. (1981) *The Culture of Public Problems: Drinking, Driving and the Symbolic Order*. Chicago: University of Chicago Press.
GWINNER, P. D. V. and GRANT, M. (1979) *What's Your Poison?* London: BBC.
HANCOCK, G. and CARIM, E. (1986) *AIDS: The Deadly Epidemic*. London: Gollancz.
HARPWOOD, D. (1982) *Tea and Tranquillisers*. London: Virago.
HARTNOLL, R. (1985) *The Nature and Extent of Drug Problems in London*. Birkbeck College, London: Drug Indicators Project.

HARTNOLL, R., DAVIAUD, I., LEWIS, R. and MITCHESON, M. (1985) *Drug Problems: Assessing Local Need (A Practical Manual for Assessing the Nature and Extent of Problematic Drug Use in a Community)*. London: Drug Indicators Project.

HARTNOLL, R., LEWIS, R., MITCHESON, M. *et al.* (1985) 'Estimating the prevalence of opioid dependence'. *Lancet*, 1, pp. 203–209.

HAW, S. (1985) *Drug Problems in Greater Glasgow*. London: Chamelion Press.

HEALTH AND SAFETY COUNCIL. (1982) *The Problem Drinker at Work*. HSE occasional paper series: OPI. London: HMSO.

HEATHER, N. and ROBERTSON, I. (1981) *Controlled Drinking*. London: Methuen.

HEATHER, N. and ROBERTSON, I. (1986) *Problem Drinking*. Harmondsworth: Pelican.

HEBDIDGE, D. (1979) *Subculture: The Meaning of Style*. London: Methuen.

HENMAN, A., LEWIS, R. and MALYON, T. (1985) *Big Deal: The Politics of the Illicit Drugs Business*. London: Pluto.

HIGGITT, A. C., LADER, M. H. and FONAGY, P. (1985) 'Clinical management of benzodiazepine dependence'. *British Medical Journal*, 291, pp. 688–690.

HINDMARCH, I. (1972) 'Adolescent drug use'. *Synapse: Journal of Edinburgh University Medical School*, 21 (3) April.

HINDMARCH, I. (1972) 'The patterns of drug abuse among school children'. *Bulletin on Narcotics*, 24, pp. 23–26.

HINGSON, R. (1983) 'FAS-like symptoms seen in pot-smokers newborn?' *The Journal*, 1st January: 2.

HINGSON, R., SCOTCH, N. A., SORENSON, J. and SWAZEY, J. P. (1981) *In Sickness and In Health*. St Louis: C. V. Mosby Company.

HOME OFFICE. (1985) *Statistics of the Misuse of Drugs in the United Kingdom*. London: Home Office.

HOME OFFICE. (1985) *Statistics of the Misuse of Drugs in the United Kingdom*. Supplementary Tables 1984. London: Government Statistical Service.

HOME OFFICE. (1986) *Tackling Drug Misuse: A Summary of the Government's Strategy*. London: Home Office.

HORE, B. D. and PLANT, M. (eds) (1980) *Alcohol Problems in Employment*. London: Croom Helm.

HORGAN, M. M., SPARROW, M. D. and BRAZEAN, R. (1986) *Alcoholic Beverage Taxation and Control Policies*. Ottawa: Brewers Association of Canada.

HUXLEY, A. (1972) *The Doors of Perception and Heaven and Hell*. Harmondsworth: Penguin.

INGLIS, B. (1975) *The Forbidden Game: A Social History of Drugs*. London: Hodder and Stoughton.

INGLIS, B. (1981) *The Diseases of Civilization*. London: Paladin.

INSTITUTE FOR THE STUDY OF DRUG DEPENDENCE. (1983) *Surveys and Statistics of Drug Taking in Britain*. London: Institute for the Study of Drug Dependence.

INTERNATIONAL LABOUR ORGANISATION. (1977) *Year Book of Labour Statistics*. 1977, 3rd Issue. Geneva: ILO.

ISRAEL, Y., GLASER, F. B., KALANT, H. *et al.* (eds) (1978) *Research Advances in Alcohol and Drug Problems*. Vol. 4. London: Plenum.

IVERSEN, L. L., IVERSEN, S. D. and SNYDEN, S. H. (eds) (1978) *Handbook of Psychopharmacology, Vol. 12, Drugs of Abuse*. London: Plenum.

IVES, R. (ed.) (1986) *Solvent Misuse in Context*. London: National Children's Bureau.

JACOBSON, B. (1981) *The Ladykillers: Why Smoking is a Feminist Issue*. London: Pluto.

JAHODA, G. and CRAMOND, J. (1972) *Children and Alcohol: A Developmental Study in Glasgow*. Vol 1. London: HMSO.

JAMES I (England) VI (Scotland) (1604) *Counterblaste to Tobacco*. London.

JAMIESON, A., GLANZ., A. and MACGREGOR, S. (1984) *Dealing with Drug Misuse*. London: Tavistock.

JOHNS, M. W. (1977) 'Self-poisoning with barbiturates in England and Wales'. *British Medical Journal*, 1, pp. 1128–30.

JOHNSON, B. D. (1973) *Marihuana Users and Drug Subcultures*. London: Wiley.

JOHNSTON, L. D., O'MALLEY, P. M. and BACHMAN, J. G. (1984) *Drugs and American High School Students 1975–1983*. National Institute on Drug Abuse, US Department of Health and Human Services, Public Health Service, Alcohol Drug Abuse and Mental Health Administration.

JUDSON, M. (1974) *Heroin Addiction in Britain*. New York: Harcourt Brace Jovanovich.

KALANT, O. J. (ed.) (1980) *Alcohol and Drug Problems in Women*. New York: Plenum.

KALB, M. (1975) 'The myth of alcoholism prevention'. *Preventative Medicine*, 4, pp. 404–416.

KANDEL, D. B. (1978) *Longitudinal Research on Drug Use*. New York: Halstead.

KANDELL, D. B. (1982) 'Epidemiological and psychosocial perspectives on adolescent drug use'. *Journal of the American Academy of Child Psychiatry*, 21, pp. 328–347.

KENDELL, R. E. (1979) 'Alcoholism: a medical or a political problem?' *British Medical Journal*, 279, pp. 367–347.

KENDELL, R. E., DE ROUMANIE, M. and RITSON, E. B. (1983) 'Effect of economic changes on Scottish drinking habits'. *British Journal of Addiction*, 78, pp. 365–380.

KENDELL, R. E., DE ROUMANIE, M. and RITSON, E. B. (1983) 'Influence of an increase in excise duty on alcohol consumption and its adverse effects'. *British Medical Journal*, 287, pp. 809–811.

KEMP, I. (1986) 'Alcohol-related deaths'. *Presentation at 21st Scottish Problems Research Symposium*, Pitlochry.

KILICH, S. and PLANT, M. A. (1980) 'Regional variations in the levels of alcohol-related problems in Britain'. *British Journal of Addiction*, 76, pp. 47–62. Also erratum 1982, 77, 211.

KINDER, B. N., PAPE, N. E. and WALFISH, S. (1980) 'Drug and alcohol education programmes: a review of outcome studies'. *International Journal of the Addictions*, 15, pp. 1035–1054.

KOOP, C. E. (1986) 'The campaign against smokeless tobacco'. *New England Medical Journal*, 314, pp. 1042–1044.

KOSVINER, A., HAWKS, D. and WEBB, M. G. T. (1973) 'Cannabis use amongst British university students. I Prevalence rates and differences between students who have tried cannabis and those who have never tried it'. *British Journal of Addiction*, 69, pp. 35–60.

KOSVINER, A. and HAWKS, D. (1977) 'Cannabis use amongst British university students. II Patterns of use and attitudes to use'. *British Journal of Addiction*, 72, pp. 41–58.

KREITMAN, N. (ed.) (1977) *Parasuicide*. Chichester: Wiley.

KREITMAN, N. (1982) 'The perils of abstention?' *British Medical Journal*, 285, pp. 444.

KREITMAN, N. (1986) 'Alcohol consumption and the preventive paradox'. *British Journal of Addiction*, 81, pp. 353–364.

LACEY, R. and WOODWARD, S. (1985) *That's Life Survey on Tranquillisers*. London: BBC.

LADER, M. (1981) 'Epidemic in the making: benzodiazepine dependence'. In: TOGNONI, G.,

BELLANTUONO, C. and LADER, M. (eds). *Epidemiological Impact of Psychotropic Drugs.* Amsterdam: Ebevier/North Holland Biomedical Press.

LADER, M. (1986) 'Management of benzodiazepine dependence – update 1986'. *British Journal of Addiction*, 81, pp. 7–10.

LADER, M. H. (1983) 'Insomnia and short-acting benzodiazepines hypnotics'. *Journal of Clinical Psychiatry*, 44, pp. 47–53.

LADER, M. H. (1983) 'Dependence on benzodiazepines'. *Journal of Clinical Psychiatry*, 44, pp. 121–127.

LADER, M. H. and PETURSSON, H. (1983) 'Rational use of anxiolytic/sedative drugs'. *New Ethicals*, July, pp. 49–77.

LATCHAM, R., KREITMAN, N., PLANT, M. A. and CRAWFORD, A. (1984) 'Regional variations in alcohol-related morbidity in Britain: a myth uncovered? I. Clinical surveys'. *British Medical Journal*, 289, pp. 1341–1343.

LAURIE, P. (1972) *Drugs: Medical, Psychological and Social Facts.* Harmondsworth: Pelican.

LEADING ARTICLE (1985) 'Media drugs campaigns may be worse than a waste of money'. *British Medical Journal*, 290, p. 416.

LECK, P., MCEWAN, J., MORETON, W. et al. (1985) *Action on Smoking at Work.* London: Academic Department of Community Medicine, King's College School of Medicine and Dentistry.

LEE, P. N. (ed.) (1976) *Statistics on Smoking in the United Kingdom.* Research Paper 1, 7th Ed. London: Tobacco Research Council.

LEWIS, R., HARTNOLL, R., BRYER, S., DAVIAUD, E. and MITCHESON, M. (1985) 'Scoring smack: the illicit heroin market in London 1980–1983'. *British Journal of Addiction*, 80, pp. 281–290.

LISHMAN, J. (ed.) (1985) *Approaches to Addiction.* London: Kogan Page.

LORD, R. (1985) *Controlled Drugs, Law and Practice.* London: Butterworths.

MCALISTER, A., PERRY, C., KILLEN, J., SLINKARD, L. A. and MAUDSY, N. (1981) 'Pilot study of smoking, alcohol and drug abuse prevention'. *American Journal of Public Health*, 70, pp. 719–725.

MCCALL SMITH, E. and MCCALL SMITH, A. (1986) *So You Want to Try Drugs.* Edinburgh: Chambers.

MCDONNELL, R. E. and MAYNARD, A. (1985) 'The costs of alcohol misuse'. *British Journal of Addiction*, 80, pp. 27–36.

MCKAY, A. J., HAWTHORNE, V. M. and MCCARTNEY, H. N. (1973) 'Drugtaking among medical students at Glasgow University'. *British Medical Journal*, 1, pp. 540–543.

MARKS, J. (1978) *The Benzodiazepines: Use, Overuse, Misuse, Abuse.* Lancaster: MTP.

MARSH, C. (1986) 'Medicine and the media'. *British Medical Journal*, 292, p. 895.

MEDICAL RESEARCH COUNCIL. (1983) *Annual Report April 1982–March 1983.* London: Medical Research Council.

MELVILLE, A. and JOHNSON, C. (1982) *Cured to Death: The Effects of Prescribed Drugs.* London: Secker and Warburg.

MERRILL, E. (1978) *Glue-Sniffing.* Birmingham: PEPAR Publications.

MIDWEEK. (1973) *Survey of Drug Use in the United Kingdom.* Social Research Design Consultancy.

MILLER, J. D., CISIN, G. H., GARDNER-KEATON, H. et al. (1983) *US National Survey on Drug Abuse: Main Findings.* National Institute on Drug Abuse, Department of Health and Human Services, Alcohol, Drug and Mental Health Administration.

MILLER, W. R. and MUNOZ, R. F. (1976) *How to Control Your Drinking*. Englewood Cliffs, New Jersey: Prentice-Hall Inc.

MILLS, P. R., LESINSKAS, D. and WATKINSON, G. (1979) 'The danger of hallucinogenic mushrooms'. *Scottish Medical Journal*, 24, pp. 316–317.

MITCHELL, A. R. H. (1972) *Drugs: The Parents' Dilemma*. London: Priory.

MORGAN, H. G. (1979) *Death Wishes? The Understanding and Management of Deliberate Self-Harm*. Chichester: Wiley.

MOTT, J. (1976) 'The epidemiology of self-reported drug misuse in the United Kingdom'. *Bulletin on Narcotics*, 28, pp. 43–54.

MOTT, J. (1985) 'Self-reported cannabis use in Great Britain in 1981'. *British Journal of Addiction*, 80, pp. 30–43.

MURRAY, R., GHODSE, H., HARRIS, C., WILLIAMS, D. and WILLIAMS, P. (eds) (1981) *The Misuse of Psychotropic Drugs*. Special Publication 1. London: Gaskell.

MYERS, T. (1982) *Alcohol and Crimes of Inter-Personal Violence*. University of Edinburgh, Ph.D. thesis.

NAHAS, G. G. (1979) *Keep off the Grass*. New York: Pergamon.

NAHAS, G. G. and PATON, W. D. M. (eds) (1979) *Marihuana Biological Effects. Analysis, Metabolism, Cellular Responses, Reproduction and Brain*. London: Pergamon.

NELSON, D. (1980) 'Mushroom magic'. *New Society*, 58, pp. 137–138.

NEWSWEEK. (1986) 'Kids and Cocaine'. March 31st, 40–45.

NOP MARKET RESEARCH LTD. (1982) Survey of drug use in the 15–21 age group undertaken for the Daily Mail. London: NOP.

O'BRIEN, C. P. (1986) 'Psychopharmacology of drug abuse'. In: DEROGATIS, L. R. (ed.), *Clinical Psychopharmacology*. Menlo Park, California: Addison-Wesley.

O'CONNOR, D. (1983) *Glue Sniffing and Volatile Substance Abuse*. Aldershot: Gower.

O'CONNOR, J. (1978) *The Young Drinkers*. London: Tavistock.

O'CONNOR, J. and DALY, M. (1985) *The Smoking Habit*. Dublin: Gill and Macmillan.

O'DONOHUE and RICHARDSON, S. (eds) (1984) *Pure Murder*. Dublin: Women's Press.

OFFICE OF POPULATION CENSUSES AND SURVEYS. (1972) *Public Attitudes to Drug-Taking*. London: Home Office Research Unit.

OFFICE OF POPULATION CENSUSES AND SURVEYS. (1978) *Occupational Mortality 1970–1972*. Decennial Supplement, Government Statistical Office. London: HMSO.

OFFICE OF POPULATION CENSUSES AND SURVEYS. (1979) *OPCS Monitor GHS*. 79/2 (August). London: HMSO.

OFFICE OF POPULATION CENSUSES AND SURVEYS. (1980) *General Household Survey 1978*. London: HMSO.

OFFICE OF POPULATION CENSUSES AND SURVEYS. (1983) *General Household Survey: Cigarette smoking 1972–1982*. London: HMSO.

OFFICE OF POPULATION CENSUSES AND SURVEYS. (1984) *General Household Survey 1982*. London: HMSO.

OFFICE OF POPULATION CENSUSES AND SURVEYS. (1985) *Drinking and Attitudes to Licensing in Scotland*. London: Government Statistical Services (OPCS Monitor SS 85/2).

OFFICE OF POPULATION CENSUSES AND SURVEYS. (1986) *Occupational Mortality 1979–80, 1982–83*, Decennial Supplement, Part 1 Commentary. London: HMSO.

ORFORD, J. (1985) *Excessive Appetites: A Psychological View of Addictions*. Chichester: Wiley.

PARKER, H., BAKX, K. and NEWCOMBE, R. (1986) *Drug Use in Wirral: The First Report of the*

Wirral Misuse of Drugs Project. Sub-department of Social Work Studies, University of Liverpool.

PATTISON, C. J., BARNES, E. A. and THORLEY, A. (1982) *South Tyneside Drug Prevalence and Indicator Study*. Newcastle: Centre for Alcohol and Drug Studies.

PATTON, C. (1985) *Sex and Germs: The Politics of AIDS*. Boston: South End Press.

PEARSON, G., GILMAN, M. and MCIVER, S. (1985) *Young People and Heroin Use in the North of England*. A report to the Health Education Council.

PECK, D. F. (1982) 'Problem drinking: some determining factors'. In: PLANT, M. A. (ed.) *Drinking and Problem Drinking*. London: Junction/Fourth Estate.

PECK, D. F. and PLANT, M. A. (1986) 'Unemployment and illegal drug use; concordant evidence from a prospective study and from national trends'. *British Medical Journal*, 293, pp. 929–932.

PEDEN, N. R. and PRINGLE, S. D. (1982) 'Hallucinogenic fungi'. *Lancet*, 1, (8268), pp. 396–392.

PETURSSON, H. J. and LADER, M. (1981) 'Benzodiazepines dependence'. *British Journal of Addiction*, 76, pp. 133–145.

PICARDIE, J. and WADE, D. (1985) *Heroin: Chasing the Dragon*. Harmondsworth: Penguin.

PICKENS, K. (1983) 'Drug education: The effects of giving information'. *Journal of Drug Education*, 13, pp. 32–44.

PITTMAN, D. J. and SYNDER, C. R. (eds) (1962) *Society, Culture and Drinking Patterns*. New York: Wiley.

PLANT, M. A. (1979) *Drugtakers in an English Town*. London: Tavistock.

PLANT, M. A. (1979) *Drinking Careers*. London: Tavistock.

PLANT, M. A. (ed.) (1982) *Drinking and Problem Drinking*. London: Junction/Fourth Estate.

PLANT, M. A. (1985) 'Alcohol in Britain: patterns, problems, paradoxes and public policy'. In: SINGLE, E. and STORM, T. (eds) *Public Drinking and Public Policy*. Toronto: Addiction Research Foundation.

PLANT, M. A., EDWARDS, G. and LADEWIG, D. (1986) *Prevention and Treatment of Drug Misuse*. Background Paper for Conference of Ministers of Health on Narcotic and Psychotropic Drug Misuse, London, 18–20 March. Geneva: World Health Organization.

PLANT, M. A., PECK, D. F. and SAMUEL, E. (1985) *Alcohol, Drugs and School-Leavers*. London: Tavistock.

PLANT, M. A. and REEVES, C. E. (1973) 'Social characteristics of drug-takers in two English urban areas'. *Drugs and Society*, 2, pp. 14–18.

PLANT, M. A. (1985) *Women, Drinking and Pregnancy*. London: Tavistock.

POLICH, J., ARMOR, D. and BRAIKER, H. (1981) *The Course of Alcoholism: 4 Years after Treatment*. New York: Wiley.

POLLOCK, S. H. (1976) 'Liberty caps: recreational hallucinogenic mushrooms' *Drug and Alcohol Dependence*, 1, pp. 445–447.

PROUDFOOT, A. T. and PARK, J. (1978) 'Changing patterns of drugs used for self-poisoning'. *British Medical Journal*, 1, pp. 90–3.

RAISTRICK, D. and DAVIDSON, R. (1985) *Alcoholism and Drug Addiction*. Edinburgh: Churchill Livingstone.

RAW, M. (1978) 'The treatment of cigarette dependence'. In: ISRAEL, Y., GLASER, F. ., KALANT, H. et al. (eds) *Research Advances in Alcohol and Drug Dependence*. Vol 4. London: Plenum.

APPENDIX II

REEVES, C. E. (1972) *Motivation for Changing Patterns of Drugtaking*. Paper presented to 30th International Congress on Alcoholism and Drug Dependence, Amsterdam.

REEVES, C. E. (1973) *Sociological Aspects of Drug Taking in Southern Hampshire*. Paper presented to 2nd International Conference on Alcoholism and Drug Dependence, Liverpool.

RELEASE. (1979) *Hallucinogenic Mushrooms*. London: Release Publications Ltd.

RELEASE. (1982) *Trouble with Tranquillisers*. London: Release Publications Ltd.

RITSON, E. B. (1985) *Community Response to Alcohol-Related Problems*. Public Health Papers No. 81. Geneva: World Health Organization.

ROBERTS, A., SHEPPARD, E., and WILSON, V. (eds) (1986) *Participating in Prevention*. Penarth: Youth Forum on Alcohol and Drugs, Council for Wales Voluntary Youth Services.

ROBERTS, J. J. K., ROBERTSON, J. R. and BUCKNALL, A. B. V. (1986) 'Management of problem drug users'. *The Physician*, June, pp. 853–856.

ROBERTS, K. (1983) *Youth and Leisure*. London: George Allen and Unwin.

ROBERTSON, I. and HEATHER, N. (1985) *So You Want to Cut Down Your Drinking*. Edinburgh: Scottish Health Education Group.

ROBERTSON, J. R. (1985) 'Drug users in contact with general practice'. *British Medical Journal*, 290, pp. 34–35.

ROBERTSON, J. R. (1986) Personal communication.

ROBERTSON, J. R. and BUCKNALL, A. B. V. (1985) 'Heroin users: notifications to the Home Office addicts index by general practitioners'. *British Medical Journal*, 291, pp. 111–113.

ROBERTSON, J. R., BUCKNALL, A. B. V., WELSBY, P. D. *et al.* (1986) 'Epidemic of AIDS-related (HTLV-111/LAV) infection among intravenous drug users'. *British Medical Journal*, 292, pp. 527–529.

ROBINS, L. M. (1978) 'The interaction of setting and pre-dispositions in explaining novel behaviour: drug initiations before, in and after Vietnam'. In: KANDEL, D. B. (ed.) *Longitudinal Research on Drug Use*, see above.

ROBINSON, D. (1979) *Talking Out of Alcoholism: The Self Help Process of Alcoholics Anonymous*. London: Croom Helm.

ROOM, R. (1977) 'Measurement and distribution of drinking patterns and problems in general populations'. In: EDWARDS, G., GROSS, H. M., KELLER, M., MOSER, J. and ROOM, R. (eds) *Alcohol-Related Disabilities*. Geneva: World Health Organization.

ROSENBAUM, M. (1981) *Women on Heroin*. Rutgers University Press.

ROSETT, H. L. and WEINER, L. (1984) *Alcohol and the Fetus*. New York: Oxford.

ROSS, H. L. (1982) *Deterring the Drinking Driver*. Lexington, Mass: Lexington Books.

ROYAL COLLEGE OF PHYSICIANS. (1971) *Smoking and Health Now*. London: Pitman.

ROYAL COLLEGE OF PHYSICIANS. (1977) *Smoking and Health*. London: Pitman Medicine.

ROYAL COLLEGE OF PHYSICIANS. (1983) *Health or Smoking?* London: Pitman.

ROYAL COLLEGE OF PSYCHIATRISTS. (1979) *Alcohol and Alcoholism*. London: Tavistock.

ROYAL COLLEGE OF PSYCHIATRISTS. (1986) *Alcohol: Our Favourite Drug*. London: Tavistock.

ROYAL LIFE SAVING SOCIETY. (1984) *Drownings in the British Isles 1983*. Studley: Royal Life Saving Society.

RUSSELL, M. A. H. (1974) 'The smoking habit and its classification'. *The Practitioner*, 212, pp. 791–800.

SANDLER, D. P., WILCOX, A. J. and EVERSON, R. B. (1985) 'Cumulative effects of lifetime passive smoking on cancer risk'. *Lancet*, 8424, pp. 312–314.

SARGENT, M. (1979) *Drinking and Alcoholism in Australia: A Power Relations Theory.* Cheshire: Longman.

SCARPITTI, F. R. and DATESMAN, S. K. (eds) (1980) *Drugs and Youth Culture.* Beverly Hills: Sage.

SCHAPS, E., DIBARTOLO, R., MOSKOWITZ, J., BALLEY, C. G. and CHURGIN, G. (1981) 'A review of 127 drug abuse prevention programme evaluations'. *Journal of Drug Issues*, 11, pp. 17–43.

SCHOFIELD, M. (1971) *The Strange Case of Pot.* Harmondsworth: Pelican.

SCOTTISH HEALTH EDUCATION CO-ORDINATING COMMITTEE. (1985) *Health Education in the Prevention of Alcohol-Related Problems.* Edinburgh: Scottish Health Education Co-ordinating Committee.

SCOTTISH HEALTH EDUCATION GROUP. (1986) *Drugs and Young People in Scotland.* Edinburgh: Scottish Health Education Group.

SCOTTISH HOME AND HEALTH DEPARTMENT. (1986) *Scottish Health Statistics 1984.* Edinburgh: HMSO.

SIMPSON, D. D. (1986) 'Addiction careers: etiology, treatment and 12-year follow-up outcomes'. *Journal of Drug Issues*, 16, pp. 107–122.

SMART, R. G. (1976) *The New Drinkers: Teenage Use and Abuse of Alcohol.* Toronto: Addiction Research Foundation.

SMART, R. G., ADLAF, E. M. and GOODSTADT, M. S. (1986) 'Alcohol and other drug use amongst Ontario students: an update'. *Canadian Journal of Public Health*, 77, pp. 57–58.

SMITH, R. (1985) 'Gissa job: the experience of unemployment'. *British Medical Journal*, 291, pp. 1263–1266.

SOLOMAN, D. and ANDREWS, G. (eds) (1973) *Drugs and Sexuality.* London: Panther.

STIMSON, G. V. (1973) *Heroin and Behaviour.* London: Irish University Press.

STIMSON, G. V. (1981) 'Epidemiological research on drug use in general populations'. In: EDWARDS, G. and BUSCH, C. (eds) *Drug Problems in Britain.* London: Academic Press.

STIMSON, G. V. and OPPENHEIMER, E. (1982) *Heroin Addiction.* London: Tavistock.

STIMSON, G. V., OPPENHEIMER, E. and THORLEY, A. (1978) 'Seven year follow-up of heroin addicts: drug use and outcome'. *British Medical Journal*, 1, 6121, pp. 1190–2.

SWISHER, J. D. (1971) 'Drug education: pushing or preventing?' *Peabody Journal of Education*, pp. 68–79.

TAYLOR, P. (1984) *Smoke Ring: The Politics of Tobacco.* London: Bodley Head.

TETHER, P. and ROBINSON, D. (1986) *Preventing Alcohol Problems.* London: Tavistock.

THOMSON, E. L. (1978) 'Smoking education programmes 1960–1976'. *American Journal of Public Health*, 68, pp. 250–251.

THORLEY, A. (1981) 'Longitudinal studies of drug dependence'. In: EDWARDS, G. and BUSCH, C. (eds) *Drug Problems in Britain.* London: Academic Press.

THORNTON, R. E. (ed.) (1978) *Smoking Behaviour.* Edinburgh: Churchill Livingstone.

THURMAN, C. (1986) Personal Communication. Adapted from Produktschap Voor Gedistilleerde Dranken (1971, 1981, 1984) *Hoeveel Alcoholhandencde Dranken Worden en in de Wereld Gedronken?* Schiedam, Netherlands.

TOBACCO ADVISORY COUNCIL. (1986) Personal Communication.

TOWNSEND, P. (1979) *Poverty in the United Kingdom.* Harmondsworth: Penguin.

TOWNSEND, P. and DAVIDSON, N. (1982) *Inequalities in Health.* Harmondsworth: Penguin.

TREBACH, A. S. (1982) *The Heroin Solution.* New Haven: Yale University Press.

TRIMBLE, M. R. (ed.) (1983) *Benzodiazepines Divided.* Chichester: Wiley.

APPENDIX II

TYLER, A. (1986) *Street Drugs*. London: New English Library.
UNITED NATIONS. (1977) *Demographic Yearbook 1976*. New York, United Nations.
VAILLANT, G. E. (1970) 'The natural history of narcotic drug addiction'. *Seminars in Psychiatry*, 2, pp. 480–498.
VAILLANT, G. E. (1973) 'A twenty year follow-up of New York narcotic addicts'. *Archives of General Psychiatry*, 29, pp. 237–241.
VAILLANT, G. E. (1983) *The Natural History of Alcoholism*. Cambridge, Mass: Harvard University Press.
WALDORF, D. (1973) *Careers in Dope*. Englewood Cliffs, New Jersey: Prentice Hall Inc.
WALLS, H. J. and BROWNLIE, A. R. (1985) *Drink, Drugs and Driving*. London: Sweet and Maxwell.
WALSH, B. M. (1980) *Drinking In Ireland*. Dublin: Economic and Social Research Unit, Broadsheet No. 2U.
WATSON, J. M. (1979) 'Solvent abuse: a retrospective study'. *Community Medicine*, 1, pp. 153–6.
WEIL, A. (1972) *The Natural Mind*. Harmondsworth: Penguin.
WELLS, B. (1973) *Psychedelic Drugs*. Harmondsworth: Penguin.
WEST, D. J. (ed.) (1978) *Problems of Drugs Abuse in Britain*. Cambridge: Institute of Criminology.
WIENER, R. S. P. (1970) *Drugs and Schoolchildren*. London: Longman.
WILLIAMS, M. (1986) 'The Thatcher generation'. *New Society*, 21st February, pp. 312–315.
WILSON, P. (1980a) *Drinking in England and Wales*. London: HMSO.
WILSON, P. (1980b) 'Drinking habits in the United Kingdom'. *Population Trends*, 22, pp. 14–18.
WORLD HEALTH ORGANISATION. (1977) *World Health Statistical Annual*. Vital Statistics and Causes of Death. Geneva: World Health Organisation.
WORLD HEALTH ORGANISATION. (1979) *Controlling the Smoking Epidemic*. Report of the WHO Expert Committee on Smoking Control, Technical Report Series 636. Geneva: World Health Organisation.
WORLD HEALTH ORGANISATION. (1984) *World Health Statistics Annual*. Geneva: World Health Organisation.
WORLD HEALTH ORGANISATION. (1985) *World Health Statistics Annual*. Geneva: World Health Organisation.
WRIGHT, J. D. (1976) 'Knowledge and experience of young people regarding drug abuse between 1969 and 1974'. *Medicine, Science and the Law*, 16, pp. 252–263.
WRIGHT, J. D. and PEARL, L. (1986) 'Knowledge and experience of young people of drug abuse 1969–84'. *British Medical Journal*, 292, p. 179.
YOUNG, J. (1971) *The Drugtakers*. London: Paladin.
YOUNG, J. and BROOKE-CRUTCHLEY, J. (1972) 'Student drug use'. *Drugs and Society*, 2, pp. 11–15.
YOUNG, R. E., MILROY, R. HUTCHISON, G. *et al.* (1982) 'The rising price of mushrooms'. *Lancet*, 1 (8269), pp. 213–214.
ZACUNE, J. and HENSMAN, C. (1971) *Drugs, Alcohol and Tobacco in Britain*. London: Heinemann.

Index

Aaro, L. E. 132
abstinence:
　syndrome 13
acquired immune deficiency
　　syndrome (*see* AIDS)
acupuncture 125
addiction: 6
　definition 7–8
addicts, recorded by Home Office 8
advertising 7, 127, 131
Advisory Council on the Misuse of
　　Drugs 134
age: 35
　and drinking 65
　and illicit drugtaking 71
　and prescribed drugs 81
　and smoking 68
AIDS 6, 27, 117, 137
Albyn House 91
alcohol:
　consumption patterns 60–65, 88–9
　description 14–17
　and the law 52–5
　related problems 15–17, 86–96,
　　120–21
alcoholic (*see* problem drinker)
Alcoholics Anonymous 4, 84, 87, 93,
　　120, 126
alcoholism:
　definition 15
alienation 43–44
amotivational syndrome 20
amphetamines:
　description 27–9
　sulphate 29

Angel dust (*see* PCP)
anomie 43–4
antibiotics 12
appetitive behaviour 9
Armor, D. J. 120
aspirins 114
Ativan 23, 80–81
autobiographical accounts
　60
availability 40–41, 93, 137–8

bad trip (*see* LSD)
Bakx, K., 75–6
Balley, C. G. 131
Bandy, P. 131
barbiturates: 80–81
　description 24–5
basic need 36
benzodiazepines: 23–4, 80–81
　description 23–4
Berridge, V. 26
Bindeman, S. 74
Binnie, H. L. 73
biological theories 33
Bostock, Y. 69–70
Brain Committee 46
brain damage 16, 121
breathalyser (*see* Lion
　　Auto-Alcometer)
Breeze, E. 63, 190–91
Brende, J. O. 123
Brewers' Society 89
British Crime Survey 74
British system 45–6
bronchitis 18, 96

Bruland, E.   132
Bucknall, A. B. V.   76, 124
Buddhism   125
Bunnie, J. E.   74
Burroughs, W.   60

Camberwell   62
cancer:
  lung   17, 98–9
cannabis:
  description   18–20
  oil   19
  resin   19
Cartwright, A. K. J.   64
Central Policy Review Staff   88
Chambers, G.   74
chasing the dragon   26
Cheltenham   77
children   27, 52, 53–4, 71
Churgin, G.   131
cigarettes   (*see* tobacco)
Clayson Committee   52–3
clinical studies   32–40, 88–90, 107–17, 118–26
coal miners   98–9
coca   1, 30
cocaine   30–31
Cohen, S.   5
Concept houses   125
constitutional theories   33
contraceptives   100
control measures   137–9
controlled drinking   120–21
Controlled Drugs Penalties Act   (1985)   47
cost   (*see* price)
councils on alcoholism   88
crack (rock)   30–31
Crawford, A.   63, 90
crime statistics   87–90
Criminal Justice (Scotland) Act (1980)   55, 91
Crowley, A.   60
CURB   25, 56
curiosity   36
Customs and Excise   103, 137

DTs   (*see* delirium tremens)

Dangerous Drugs Act (1920)   45
Dangerous Drugs (Prevention of Misuse) Act (1967)   46
Davidson, R.   124
Davies, J.   69–70
de Alarcon, R.   75
deaths   (*see* mortality)
Defence of the Realm Act (1916)   45
delinquency   40
delirium tremens   13, 16
Department of Health and Social Security   80–81
dependence: 13, 15
  definition   13
de Roumanie, M.   63
designer drugs   27
deviance   5, 44
Dexedrine   27
Dibartolo, R.   131
Diconal   26, 109, 112
Dight, S.   64–5
disease model   15–16, 120
Divine Light Mission   125
doctors   40, 92, 98–100
Dorn, N.   131
Doyle, C.   117
drinking habits:
  in Britain   60–61, 63–5
  in different countries   61–2
Drinkwatchers   88
drowning   88
drug:
  definition   12
  offences   81
drugtakers:
  general   70–79
  known to agencies   103–15
Drug Trafficking Offences Act (1986)   51
drunken driving   54–5, 89, 138
drunkenness:
  and the law   54–5, 88–90
Duffy, J.   53, 93
Dunlop Committee   55
Dyer, J.   113

Ecstasy   21
Edinburgh   27, 76, 114

INDEX

educational problems 37–8
Edwards, G. 1–2, 5, 64, 124
Electoral Register 59–60
Elwood, J. M. 132
emphysema 16
endorphines 33
England 62–4, 69–70
environmental theories 37–42
Erroll Committee 52
escalation 118, 126

family disturbance 37
Family Expenditure Survey 59
Finland 138
First International Opium Convention (1912) 45
Fish, F. 74
fishermen 92
fits 16
flashbacks 22
fly agaric 21
foetal alcohol syndrome 16–17, 95
freebasing 30–31

gambling 9
gastritis 16
Ghodse, H. 114, 124
Gillies, P. 132
Glanz, R. 107, 124
Glaser, D. 131
Glasgow 75
glues:
    description 22–3
Goode, E. 77, 79

hallucinogens 20–22, 29–30
hangovers 14
Hartnoll, R. 76
hashish (*see* cannabis)
Hauknes, A. 132
Haw, S. 75
Hawks, D. 74
Hawthorne, V. M. 74
health education 127–37, 139, 141
Health Education Council 127–9
heart disease 17, 23
Heather, N. N. 120
hedonism 35

hepatitis 27
heroin 25–7
Hindmarch, I. 74
historical factors 42–3
HIV (*see* AIDS)
Home Office 89, 103
homosexuality 9, 117
Huxley, A. 21, 60
hydrocarbons (*see* glues)

ideology 39–40, 72
illicit drugtakers:
    age 35
    sex 34
    social class 38
illicit drugtaking:
    prevalence 70–9
immigration 42
individual theories 33–7
industrial costs 84
injection 13
intelligence 34
Intoxicating Substances (Supply) Act (1985) 47
Ipswich experiment 28, 41
Iran 5
Islam 10, 40

James VI and I 17
Jamieson, A. 124
Johns, M. W. 114
joint 19, 29
Jordan, M. M. 74
junkie 111

Kalb, M. 131
Kemp, I. 91
Kendell, R. E. 63, 88
Killen, J. 132
Kinder, B. N. 131
Kosviner, A. 74
Kreitman, N. 90, 113

LSD:
    description 20–22
    trip 21
Lader, M. H. 24, 116
Latcham, R. 90

laudanum 25
law 45–57
learning to drink 65
Leary, T. 60
Leck, P. 66
Legalise Cannabis Campaign 10, 84
Liberty Cap mushrooms 21, 57
Librium 23–4, 180–81
Licensing (Scotland) Act (1976) 53
Lion Auto-Alcometer 54
liquor licensing laws 52–3
liver cirrhosis 7, 16, 85, 88–9, 92–4
Lochsen, P. M. 132
lung cancer (*see* cancer)

MDA 21
MDMA (*see* Ecstasy)
MORI 79
Macgregor, S. 124
Mandrax 25
marijuana (marihuana) (*see* cannabis)
Marks, J. 79
Marsh, C. 134
Maudsy, N. 132
Maynard, A. 84
McAlister, A. 132
McCartney, H. M. 74
McDonnell, R. 84
McEwan, J. 66
McKay, A. M. 74
Medicines Act (1968) 56
Medicines Commission 55
Medicines (Prescriptions Only) Amendment (No. 2) Order (1978) 57
Medicines (Prescriptions Only) Order (1977) 57
men (*see* sex differences)
Merseyside, Cheshire and Lancashire Council on Alcoholism 93
mescalin 21
Methadone 26–7
Methaqualone (*see* Mandrax)
Methedrine 29
Miller, W. R. 120
Misuse of Drugs Act (1971) 47–50, 56, 85, 103–7
Misuse of Drugs Act (1971)

Modification Order (1985) 47
Moreton, W. 66
morphine 25–7
mortality:
  liver cirrhosis 89–96
  tobacco-related 7, 17–18
Moskowitz, J. 131
Mott, J. 74
Munoz, R. F. 120
Murdock, G. 73

national differences:
  in alcohol problems 93–5
  in drinking habits 62
  in tobacco problems 100–102
Newcombe, R. 75–6
Newsweek 31
Nicot, J. 17
nicotine 17
non-response 59–60
NOP Market Research Ltd 74–5
Northern Ireland 63, 69–70
Norway 138
notified addicts 107–9
nurses 40, 100
nutmeg 31

occupation:
  and alcohol problems 40, 91–3
  and drug problems 40
  and lung cancer 98–9
Office of Population Censuses and Surveys 67–9, 92, 97–8
opiates:
  description 25–7
opium 25–7
opium wars 45
Oppenheimer, E. 110, 124
overdoses (*see* parasuicide)
over prescription 24

PCP: 5
  description 29–30
pancreatitis 16
Pape, N. E. 131
Paracetamol 115
parasuicide: 7, 110, 112–14
  definition 113

INDEX

Park, J. 114
Parker, H. 75–6
Parson, E. R. 123
passive smoking 102–3
Pearson, J. C. G. 132
Peck, D. F. 76, 96
peer pressure 38–9, 72–3
peptides 33
Perry, C. 132
personal problems 34–6
personality traits 33–4
Petursson, J. H. 116
peyote 1
phenothiazines 24
physical dependence: 15
  definition 13
Pickens, K. 131–2
pilots 99
Plant, M. A. 53, 63, 74, 76–7, 90, 93
Plant, M. L. 17
police powers 46–57
Polich, J. M. 120
polydrug use 77–9, 111, 114
poppyhead tea 25
pregnancy 16–17, 18, 22, 24, 27, 95, 100
President, P. A. 131
  prescriptions 79–81
price 41, 138
problem drinker:
  definition 15–16
Prohibition 41, 138
Protection of Children (Tobacco) Act (1986) 52
Proudfoot, A. T. 114
psilocybin 21
psychedelic drugs 20–22, 29–30
psychological dependence:
  definition 13
publicans 92
pushers 2–3 (see also dealers)

Raistrick, D. 124
Rathod, N. H. 75
Raw, M. 122
reefer (see joint)
Reeves, C. E. 77
refusals 60

regional variations:
  in drinking habits 63–5
  in drinking problems 90–91
  in drug use 75–6
  in smoking habits 69–70
  in tobacco-related diseases 97–8
religion 39–40
remissions 120–21, 124–5
restaurateurs 92
risk-taking 36
Ritalin 27
Ritson, E. B. 63
Road Traffic Act (1972) 54
Robertson, I. 120
Robertson, J. R. 76, 117, 124
Robins, L. 123
Rolleston Committee 45
Royal College of Physicians 65–6, 96–7, 131, 132
Royal College of Psychiatrists 84, 88, 138
Royal Lifesaving Society 88
Russell, M. A. H. 96

Sainsbury Committee 55
Samuel, E. 76
Schaps, E. 131
school pupils 59, 65, 76
Scientology 125
Scotland 52–3, 62–5, 69–70
Scottish Health Education Group 14, 127, 129, 132, 134
Scottish Home and Health Department 89
seamen 92
self-destruction 36
self-medication 35
sentencing of drug offenders 51–2, 107
sex differences: 34, 85, 93, 95
  and alcohol problems 93–5
  and drinking 63
  and drug problems 71–2
  and smoking 68
  and tobacco problems 101–2
Sheehay, M. 124
shooting galleries 27
Single Convention 46
Skid Row 88

Skoal Bandits   18
Slinkard, L. A.   132
Snow, M.   131
snuff dipping   18
social class   38, 78
social reactions   44
sociological theories   43–4
solvents   (*see* glues)
Sporting Events (Control of Alcohol Etc.) Act (1985)   55
Spratley, T. A.   64
Stambull, H. B.   120
stereotype   11
Stimson, G. V.   110–11, 124
students   73, 74, 76, 100
suicide   22, 121, 123
surveys: 59–60
  of drug problems   59, 85
  of drug use   59, 73–7, 85
Swisher, J. D.   131
Synanon   125

THC   18
Taylor, C.   107, 124
taxes on drugs   7, 140
Thalidomide   55
therapeutic addicts   5, 46
Therapeutic Substances Act (1925)   55
Thomson, E. L.   132
Thorley, A.   124
Thurman, C.   62, 89
tobacco:
  consumption of   65–70
  description   17–18
  and the law   52
  and mortality   7, 17–18
  and pregnancy   18

Tofranil   24
tolerance:
  definition   12–13, 23
toluene   23
trafficking   (*see* dealers)
tranquillisers   23–4, 47, 81, 115–17
transcendental meditation   125
Transport Act (1981)   54
treatment   125–6
Triptizol   24
tuberculosis   16

ulcers   16
under-reporting   59
unemployment   10, 37–8, 75–6

validity   59–60
Valium   23–4, 80–81
Vietnam War   28, 123

Wales   52–3
Walfish, S.   131
Wells, B. W. P.   74
Wiener, R. S. P.   74
Willcox, B.   132
Williams, M.   76
Wilson, P.   63
Wirral   75–6
withdrawal symptoms   13–14, 24, 26–7
women   (*see* sex differences)
Wootton Report   47
World Health Organization   94, 97, 99

young people:
  in licensed premises   53–4